Curing Diabetes in 7 Steps

• • • • • • •

Take control of, and reverse your type two diabetes using Functional Medicine, naturally

Laurens Maas
B.Sc. Ost. Dl.Hom.
G.Os.C & FBIH (UK)

Curing Diabetes in 7 Steps: Take control of, and reverse your type two diabetes using Functional Medicine, naturally

Copyright © 2013 Laurens Maas. All rights reserved. No part of this book may be reproduced or retransmitted in any form or by any means without the written permission of the publisher.

Published by Wheatmark®
1760 East River Road, Suite 145
Tucson, Arizona 85718 U.S.A.
www.wheatmark.com

ISBN: 978-1-60494-397-9
LCCN: 2009942294

"What I've learned from God personally is that as soon as you get the lesson, it's over . . . that's what Grace is."

Oprah Winfrey

"Rough seas make good sailors"

Anonymous

Contents

Gratitudes .... *ix*
Medical Disclaimer .... *xi*
About the Author .... *xiii*
Foreword .... *xv*
Preface .... *xix*

Introduction 1
About Diabetes 8
Step 1: Learn about Carbohydrates 43
Step 2: Learn about Proteins 50
Step 3: Burning Fats According to Your Metabolic Type 59
Step 4: Learn about Minerals 87
Step 5: Stress and the Side Effects 90
Step 6: Learn about Exercise 104
Step 7: The Ultimate Goal—Stabilize the Blood Glucose and
    Insulin Levels 109
Conclusion 114

Appendices *117*
    Useful Contacts *119*
    Glycemic Indexes of Selected Foods *120*
    Results, Interpretation Charts, and Treatment Guides *125*
    Shopping List *133*
    Healthy Recipes *149*

Gratitudes

Thank you to my wife, Cath, and my three children, Phoenix, Phoebe, and Cosmo; I am blessed to be with you all.

Thank you to a multitude of my diabetic patients, who helped me uncover, through careful observation and testing, how to get rid of type 2 diabetes. Thank you for allowing me to monitor your progress and for sharing your experiences with me. Without you I would not be the physician I am today.

Many thanks to Dr. Bruce Shelton MD Di.Hom., Dr. Joseph Mercola DO, Dr. Dicken Weatherby ND, and Dr. Dan Kalish DC for the knowledge and guidance they share and impart so willingly to make humanity healthy. I have found all of them to be a constant source of inspiration.

Special thanks goes to Dr. Patrick Hanaway MD, Head of Genova Labs for writing the foreword for the book in such a short space of time.

Thank you to all the scientists and staff at Genova diagnostic Labs USA for all your support during my 19 years of practice – especially with regards to your excellent diagnostic testing in helping me solve so many patients' problems.

Medical Disclaimer

All clinical material published by the author is for informational purposes only. Readers are encouraged to confirm the holistic and medical information contained herein with other references and sources.

Patients and consumers should consult their physician or health care provider before embarking on any health program such as this. This raises a good opportunity to get some blood and hormone tests done while discussing the merits of this book.

The information contained herein, is not intended to replace the medical advice offered by your physician. The author will not be liable for any direct, indirect, consequential, special, exemplary, or other damages arising there from.

About the Author

Laurens Maas B.Sc. Ost. DI Hom. G.Os.C & FBIH (UK)

Laurens Maas is a registered osteopath, nutritionist, and homeopath. He trained in the United Kingdom and the United States and has been practicing **holistic medicine** for over nineteen years. He is currently in training for his integrated Medical Doctoral degree.

In this time he has used the techniques outlined in this book to consult with, and treat, thousands of patients, including professional athletes, celebrities, pop stars, medical doctors and professors.

From his clinic in Barbados, Laurens Maas treats clients from the local Caribbean region and receives hundreds of patients who fly in from all over the world specifically for his treatment and to learn how to care for themselves using the 5 Laws. His treatment methods include state of the art, functional medicine (FM).

Foreword

Patrick Hanaway, MD
Chief Medical Officer
Genova Diagnostics

I am thrilled to contribute my respect and admiration for the incredible work that Laurens Maas has been offering to help heal people with complex, chronic disease from all around the world. Laurens now gives wisdom to all beings – especially the nearly one-third of people at risk of developing Type II Diabetes Mellitus (T2DM). The methods in this book are based upon the unique operating system known as Functional Medicine. In this case, the term *functional* is not in opposition to the dysfunctional medicine that focuses on symptom suppression with pharmaceutical agents; rather, it highlights the opportunity to FUNCTION optimally well. All too often, health is perceived as the absence of illness, but the same tools that will help to cure diseases like T2DM will also help us achieve and maintain well-being!

The Functional Medicine Matrix Model gathers subjective and objective information from the client/ patient to understand physiologic imbalances within systems of: digestion, immune modulation, energy production, elimination of waste/toxins, circulation/ transportation, and structural integrity. Therapeutic interventions focus on bringing these systems back into balance through the appropriate used of nutrition, exercise, stress reduction, sleep, and connection. These are precisely the tools that Dr. Maas utilizes in his first book (*The Hidden Cure and The Five Laws of Perfect Health*, 2009) and again in his new book as he tackles the incredible burden of disease manifesting as diabetes, metabolic syndrome, and Alzheimer's disease. Within this book are the tools to help our people.

Dr. Maas offers a straight forward and practical program to understand

and reverse the progression toward diabetes mellitus (DM). Through his writings, he first creates a visceral awareness of the magnitude of the tremendous issues with diabetes via a series of startling statistics, then moves quickly to the personal level with a provocative comparison between cocaine and sugar – forcing us to re-evaluate our relationship with sugar. Through this heightened awareness, we learn of the progression of imbalance and disease that arises from the diabetic domino effect. Fortunately, we also learn of the tools and approaches that Dr. Maas has used successfully over the past seventeen years to reverse diabetes and induce weight loss.

The steps offered here are tried and true, embodying nutritional recommendations that are personalized to meet your specific needs; to identify the optimal proportion and types of fats, proteins, and carbohydrates FOR YOU... based upon your unique metabolic type. The process of personalized (or bespoke) treatments takes your biochemical individuality into account, for we are as different in our internal metabolic pathways as we are in our external appearance. During our lifetimes we eat twenty-five to fifty tonnes of food, both macronutrients and micronutrients. It is necessary that this fuel is attuned to optimize the functioning of our metabolic machinery.

In reading this book, whose contents are familiar to me, I was impressed by the pivot point in chapter three with discussions of the hormonal pathways and relationships that impact diabetes and weight gain, as well as the deleterious, obesogenic effect of artificial hormone-like chemicals from our environment. This awareness in the assessment and treatment of both obesity and diabetes provides an expanded view of the relationship between our bodies and the environment. Here we learn about the effects of food, supplements, sleep and exercise, along with the hormones, on our metabolism.

Chapter five follows up quickly with emphasis on the role of stress and the adrenal glands in overall health and well-being. Dr. Maas demonstrates his deep understanding of the inter-relatedness of these metabolic pathways in supporting individuals on the path to wellness. There is recognition that a systems-based approach is necessary to provide the foundation for healing. This is not a process of picking one from column A and two from column B, as is seen with many other one size fits all approaches. In reality we recognize that one size fits all means that the size (or program) being offered doesn't fit *any* real person, only the fictitious average person. Again, we see the merit—in fact the necessity—of a personalized approach to our health and well-being.

The cutting edge monograph makes laser-like points about the nature of illness and healing using up-to-date analysis of the peer-reviewed literature. The information presented can help you to share this powerful approach with your health care practitioner, as you move in the direction of healing. Even experienced health care practitioners can and will learn from Laurens Maas' experience, as I did reading about Goats Rue and its relationship with the oft-prescribed metformin. Each person who opens these pages will be changed by the information, knowledge, and wisdom embodied here. I invite you to open your mind on this journey towards healing, becoming more whole, with Laurens Maas. . . and I offer great thanks to him for sharing his journey of healing with us.

Dr. Patrick Hanaway, MD
July 8, 2012

Preface

Laurens Maas has uncovered that diabetes, as well as weight-gain, heart disease and cancer, is caused by the combination of dangerous levels of yeast fermentation, excess synthetic estrogens and simple sugars in our environment. Today these three elements are abundant in our surroundings and diet at greater levels than previous generations.

Through many years of research and observing his patients, Laurens Maas has discovered that many people are unknowingly infected with a high level of internal 'fermentation' due to yeast and other fungal activity.

This is because the external and internal environments of humans today are very "fungal," or degenerative. Modern foods often contain high levels of sugar, yeast, and fermented food items which, when combined, create the conditions for fungal growth.

Not only are these foodstuffs more prevalent in modern society than in the past, but people are also consuming more of these dangerous substances than ever before. For instance, the average American today eats 140-160 lbs. of sugar per year. 300 years ago the average consumption of sugar was 3-4 lbs. per year. Diabetes was extremely rare in those days.

In addition to these foodstuffs, modern societies have a high use of antibiotics, hormones, birth control pills, hormone replacement therapies, and Obesogens, otherwise known as Endocrine Disrupting Chemicals (EDC's), all of which are detrimental to the human body. (Diamanti-Kandarakis E et al. 2009)[1]

What's more, many pesticides and pollutants behave like estrogen within

---

1 Evanthia Diamanti-Kandarakis, Jean-Pierre Bourguignon, Linda C. Giudice, Russ Hauser, Gail S. Prins, Ana M. Soto, R. Thomas Zoeller, and Andrea C. Gore. 2009 "Endocrine-Disrupting Chemicals: An Endocrine Society Scientific Statement." *Endocrine Reviews* 30(4): 293-342, doi: 10.1210/er.2009-0002

our bodies, and it is clear that people today are unwittingly consuming more of these due to estrogen and antibiotic residues working their way into our food pyramid.

This 'estrogenization' of our environment has taken its toll on the health of the population and is in some way responsible for the accelerated rates of diabetes, as well as cancer, weight-gain, heart diseases and death.

This book highlights that the main causes of diabetes in our environment are fungus, yeast, pesticides, and synthetic hormones, xenobiotics, xeno-estrogens and Obesogens. These are also combined with a serious decline in the natural metabolic hormones that help burn fat and an increase in the hormones that cause fat storage.

This book presents an effective way for you to scientifically reverse your diabetes. Each day read one chapter - this will teach you one step towards curing your diabetes. All together there are seven steps you need to follow to cure your diabetes, and therefore seven chapters in this book.

If you are new to complementary health, please read this entire book before you start the program so you can get an understanding of the seven steps. Then read it a second time applying each of the steps over an appropriate period of time such as seven weeks. Alternatively, if you are familiar with applied nutrition use the seven steps as you read through the material, applying the lessons learnt as you go. This will fast track the process.

"Over many years of daily clinical practice and patient observation, time and time again I have seen that these really are the best techniques for effectively reversing diabetes and inducing weight loss." (Laurens Maas 2009)

Curing Diabetes in 7 Steps

Introduction

This book is about a molecule that is so powerful that it will determine whether you will suffer from chronic yeast infections, heart disease, cancer, diabetes, Alzheimer's, arthritis, weight gain and many other diseases. This molecule also determines your overall longevity. It is this same molecule that will determine if your weight loss program fails or not.

The molecule we are talking about is called glucose or sugar. Unfortunately, the refined sugar molecule is very addictive. Once it is inside our bodies, it generates the release of a pleasure neurotransmitter called 'Serotonin'. Just because it feels good, it doesn't mean it's right.

This powerful molecule, found in nature, is responsible for our cellular energy. However, when over "refined and processed" this molecule can become deadly because it has been *"pharmaceuticalized"*.

Cocaine vs. Sugar. Which one is worse?

One *cannot* find pure granulated sugar in the natural world. It's always balanced with minerals and vitamins such as in fruit, ground foods and vegetables, and this helps to stabilize glucose' volatile nature.

Very similarly one *cannot* find cocaine in its pure, white powder form within nature. Cocaine is an extraction of the leaves of the *Erythroxylon coca* bush, which is indigenous to the Andean highlands of South America. As of June 15th, 2012, the US Office of National Drug Control Policy cited that a grand majority of the cocaine available in the U.S. is transported from the country of Colombia.

Chewing coca leaves does induce euphoria but does not induce addiction whereas the pharmaceutical or pure cocaine can. Cocaine is the most frequently reported illicit substance associated with drug abuse fatalities and causes three times more deaths than any other illegal drug (Platt 1997)[1].

- Also, nearly 1/3rd of the deaths linked with cocaine use are caused by the direct pharmacological effects of the drug itself.
- Nearly 35.9 million Americans aged 12 and older have tried cocaine at least once in their lifetime, according to a national survey, and about 2.1 million Americans are regular users[2].
- The vast majority of deaths related to cocaine are caused by homicide, suicide, and motor vehicle collisions as a result of the drug's mind-altering properties[3].
- There are more than two million Americans that currently use cocaine, just over 700,000 are users of freebase or crack cocaine[4].
- Cocaine kills 2,500 Americans a year.
- Cocaine is a stimulant that can cause organ failure in the heart, kidneys and lungs if taken in excessive quantities[5].
- Globally 14 million to 21 million people use cocaine[6].

So what are the facts about diabetes?

- High glucose levels in the blood are associated with a shortened lifespan and increased risk of disease.[7]
- Over 346 million people suffer from diabetes around the world and this number is forecast to get worse over the next decade[8].

---

1 Platt, Jerome J. 1997. *Cocaine Addiction: Theory, Research, and Treatment*. Cambridge, MA: Harvard University Press.
2 Ibid.
3 Ibid.
4 Ibid.
5 U.S. Department of Health and Human Services National Institutes of Health http://archives.drugabuse.gov/pdf/monographs/ - 1975-2006
6 Jeannine Stein. 2012. "200 million people use illegal drugs; what is the toll on health?" *Los Angeles Times*, January 05.
7 Leiden Longevity study (LLS) Group. *Human Insulin and IGF-1 and familial longevity at middle age, Aging, 2009 Jul 24;1(8): 714-22* - http://www.ncbi.nlm.nih.gov/pubmed/20157552
8 http://www.who.int/diabetes/en/

- Approximately 90% of people with Type 2 diabetes are obese.[9]
- Every 10 seconds someone dies from diabetes-related causes globally.
- Every year nearly 3.5 million people in the world die due to diabetes. The death rate is expected to rise by 25% over the next decade.[10]
- The World Health Organization (WHO) reports that diabetes has reached epidemic proportions and expects that 80% of all new cases of diabetes will appear in developing countries by 2025.[11]
- Individuals with diabetes are more likely to die from a heart attack than those who don't have diabetes.[12]

So what's worse, having a cocaine addiction or a sugar addiction?

Of course it is sugar, as it's responsible for many more deaths worldwide. Sugar is a legal drug. Cocaine is illegal. One must remember that T2 Diabetes is a lifestyle disease centered around sugar and as it is legal and as addictive as cocaine, its use is far more widespread. Both cocaine and sugar are bad for the body as they both induce illness and disease and ruin the fabric of society.

Our lifestyle and food choices can cause us to have, or save us from, diabetes – the choice is yours.

Can you reverse your T2 diabetes and get rid of it for good?

The answer is yes you can. You can obtain optimal blood sugar scores using diet and exercise and maybe a few natural hormones.

This book is a guide that you can apply to your day-to-day life which will help you cure your T2 diabetes. It teaches you how to use and control your diet, in order to control your diabetes.

It contains key insights that I have revealed and perfected over the years, and solutions which really work to change your sugar handling capacity.

After just one week to a month of sticking to the seven steps in this book, you will see your blood sugar handling greatly improve. When you measure your blood sugar levels you will see them begin to normalize and you will feel better and better.

---

9   Ibid.
10 *Diabetes Facts.* WorldDiabetesFoundation.org.http://www.worlddiabetesfoundation.org/composite-35.htm
11 Ibid 9.
12 William A. Petit Jr., M.D. & Adamec, Christine. 2002. *The Encyclopedia of Diabetes.* New York, NY: Facts on File.

Each chapter's lesson builds on the previous chapter's lesson and teaches you about carbohydrates, proteins, fats, minerals and your state of mind. The information contained within the pages of this short book will create a shift in your biology away from the disease of Type 2 diabetes.

You will need to be disciplined, and monitor your blood sugar measurements as you go through the steps. You will see the fasting blood sugar slowly change to become better and better.

Take one day at a time, building and getting stronger until you have completed your first week. Calculate the percentage improvement and repeat another seven day cycle until the blood sugars are as close to optimal as possible.

You'll have to monitor your changes with blood sugar measurements. One gold standard in blood chemistry is the HbA1c test, which tells you how well your blood glucose is going. We'll learn about that a little later in step seven - the monthly carbohydrate evaluation of the body.

In other words, your HbA1c will tell you how well your body's sugar handling is going over a long period of time (over months) whereas daily glucose testing tells you how your body handles sugar on a day to day, meal to meal basis.

Did you know that 66% of African / American diabetics die of heart attacks or strokes?[13]

Decades ago Type 2 Diabetes would usually be *adult*-onset but Type 2 Diabetes is such a pandemic problem now in America that younger and younger children, on a pediatric level, are being affected at an alarming rate. Below is a statement from the 2006 publication of The Council of State Governments,[14] USA.

> *Experts are also concerned that chronic diseases are appearing among younger adults, adolescents and children. For example, health care providers and the Centers for Disease Control and Prevention are finding cases of type 2 (adult onset) diabetes among children. While no national trend data yet exist, experts estimate that up to 45 percent of all new diabetes patients are*

---

13 National Diabetes Education Program- CDC (USA) http://ndep.nih.gov/resources/ResourceDetail.aspx?ResId=230

14 Michael P. Fierro, http://www.healthystates.csg.org/NR/rdonlyres/E42141D1-4D47-4119-BFF4-A2E7FE81C698/0/Trends_Alert.pdf for The Council of State Governments. 2006.

currently being identified in large pediatric centers. Twenty years ago, it was unheard of for children or adolescents to be diagnosed with type 2 diabetes.

It is the medical tragedy of our time that the medical establishment chooses to ignore the possibility that type 2 diabetes can be reversed. Hopefully this book will be a step in the right direction whereby you will start to create a better future for yourself, reverse your diabetes and avoid heart attacks and strokes.

To prevent strokes and heart attacks in diabetics the answer is not more medication, but a better diet and lifestyle (and maybe some natural hormones).

Diabetics do not die from diabetes; they die because of the consequences of diabetes such as heart disease[15]-[16]-[17], strokes[18], cancer[19], blindness[20] or kidney disease[21]. They will also suffer from weight gain or obesity, blindness and amputations.

The only real way to prevent these consequences is to treat the cause of

---

15   Coutinho M, Gerstein H, Poque J, Wang Y, Yusuf S. *The relationship between glucose and incident cardiovascular events, a meta regression analysis of published data from 20 studies of 95,783 individuals followed for 12.4 years.* Diabetes care 1999 Feb; 22(2):233-240 - http://www.ncbi.nlm.nih.gov/pubmed/10333939

16   de Vegt F, Dekker JM, Ruhe HG et al. *Hyperglycaemia is associated with all cause and cardiovascular mortality in the Hoorn population; the Hoorn Study.* Diabetologia. 199 Aug;42 (8): 926-931 - https://www.aace.com/sites/all/files/dccwhitepaper.pdf

17   Ceriello A. *Impaired glucose tolerance and CVD: the possible role of post-prandial hyperglycaemia.* Am.Heart Journal. 2004 May;147(5); 803-807-- http://www.ahjonline.com/article/S0002-8703(03)00857-3/abstract

18   Batty GD, Kivimaki M, Smith GD, Marmot MG, Shipley MJ. *Post challenge blood glucose concentration and stroke mortality rates in non-diabetic men in London UK; 38-year follow up of the original Whitehall prospective cohort study.* Diabetologia 2008 July (7): 1123-1126- http://www.ncbi.nlm.nih.gov/pmc/articles/PMC2440932/

19   Stocks T, Lukanova A, Bjorge T, et al. *Metabolic factors and the risk of colorectal cancer in 580,000 men and women in the metabolic syndrome & cancer project* (Me-Can): Metabolic Syndrome Cancer Project Group. Cancer 2010 Dec 17.-- http://onlinelibrary.wiley.com/doi/10.1002/cncr.25772/abstract

20   Cheng YJ, Gregg EW, Geiss LS, *Association of HbA1C and fasting plasma glucose levels with diabetic retinopathy prevalence n the US population; implication for diabetes diagnostic thresholds.* Diabetes Care 2009 Nov;32(11): 2027-2032-- http://care.diabetesjournals.org/content/32/11/2027.abstract?ijkey=9dc9e1bcd4be7a719da8520f6022f76e65dbe51f&keytype2=tf_ipsecsha

21   Bakris GL, *Recognition, pathogenesis and treatment of different stages of nephropathy in patients with type 2 diabetes mellitus.* Mayo Clinic Proc. 2011 May ; 86(5);444-456 -- http://www.mayoclinicproceedings.org/article/S0025-6196(11)60034-7/abstract

diabetes, which is sugar. Uncontrolled sugar consumption creates inflammation within the arteries and veins[22]. Furthermore, if you control the carbohydrates, you will control the level of inflammation or restrict the amount of vascular damage within the body.

After completing the steps in this book, my patients say that they feel cooler. Their body temperature feels as if it has lowered, but what has actually happened is that they have changed the level of inflammation within their blood vessels and tissues, giving their pancreas and body a chance to heal.

Excess sugar in the blood will easily turn into an alcohol-like effect in the blood stream, especially if there is yeast overgrowth within the body. The sugar-yeast-alcohol connection causes the body temperature to rise from systemic inflammation. More sugar equals more heat, and if it's not burned off it will heat the body (inflammation) and eventually turn to fat. The inflammation also irritates the nerves and 60-70% of people with diabetes have mild to severe forms of nervous system damage[23]. As you control your sugars, you will notice that your brain and muscles work better.

As you physically feel better, your blood chemistry will improve, reflecting the benefits of the implemented program. As you take each seven day cycle or week of the program, you will see your test results get better and better.

So enjoy the seven steps process and judge the results for yourself at the end of your first month.

If you're a skeptic then all I can ask is for you to use *science* to prove your recovery. This book tells you how to scientifically monitor your HbA1C[24] levels and evaluate your recovery as well as uncover how to cure yourself. T2 Diabetes can be managed and reversed [25,26] when you start to really treat it,

---

[22] Jackson CA, Yudkin JS, Forrest RD. *A comparison of the relationships of the glucose tolerance test and the glycated haemoglobin assay with diabetic vascular disease in the community.* The Islington Diabetes Survey. Diabetes Res Clin Pract. 1992 Aug;17(2):111–123. --http://www.ncbi.nlm.nih.gov/pubmed/1425145

[23] Diabetes Statistics, Diabetes .org; accessed April 2012.- http://www.diabetes.org/diabetes-basics/diabetes-statistics/

[24] American College of Endocrinology Consensus Statement on Guidelines for Glycemic Control – Endocrine Practice Vol 8 (Suppl 1) January/February 2002 ; 7

[25] Pehuet-Figoni M, Ballot E, Bach JF, Chatenoud L. *Aberrant function and long-term survival of mouse Beta cells exposed to in vitro to high glucose concentrations.* Cell Transplant 1994 Sep-Oct;3(5): 445-451 -http://www.ncbi.nlm.nih.gov/pubmed/7827783

[26] Gleason CE, Gonzalez M, Harmon JS, Robertson RP. *Determinants of Glucose toxicity*

which requires a thorough understanding of how diet choices have a massive impact in our overall pancreatic health and the disease condition.

As you see the daily and monthly evaluation results reflect an improvement in your pancreas, you can be sure that you're on your way to getting rid of your diabetes and restoring your body's natural handling of sugars and carbohydrates.

So let's read about what diabetes is and the recent breakthrough studies that show that it can be reversed.

---

and its revrsibilty in pancreatic islet Beta-cell line HIT-T15. Am. J Physiol Endcrinol Metab 20000;279: E 997-E1002-- http://www.ncbi.nlm.nih.gov/pubmed/11052953

About Diabetes

1. What is Diabetes?

Diabetes happens when the body loses control of its blood sugar levels, usually causing the blood to have too much sugar in it. Sugar, as a molecule, is very powerful because it has built into its structure a lot of stored energy. That energy needs to be controlled. It's like handling gasoline, you have got to be very careful how much is used otherwise, if control is lost, it can catch fire and burn. It's similar to diabetes. When sugar remains in the blood it cannot be used for energy production, because that takes place in the cells of the body. The pancreas is the organ that is responsible for controlling the blood sugar levels. As the sugar stays in the blood, outside of the cells, it's burning the insides, inflaming the vessels.

The pancreas is situated just next to and below your stomach. The key hormone that is produced by the pancreas is called insulin.

Special cells within the pancreas, called the beta cells, produce the insulin. Insulin causes the body to take the sugar *out* of the blood stream and put it *into* the cells. Insulin is similar to the gasoline pump attendant, helping to put the fuel into the cells.

If the gasoline pump attendant (insulin) doesn't do its proper job and starts to spill gasoline all over the floor, it can pollute, do damage and even catch alight. Inflammation is due to excess sugar/ excess energy and this spillage can really burn vessels, organs and nerves.

There are two forms of diabetes in humans and possibly a third that is now coming into recognition.

Type 1 diabetes *is a situation when the beta cells no longer produce any insulin.*

Of course, this type of diabetic has to use insulin to stay alive. This is a clear case of insulin deficiency. This is usually diagnosed in children and young adults and they must manage this kind of diabetes with daily insulin injections. The cause of type 1 diabetes is usually due to the immune system attacking the pancreas, typically as the result of a virus or autoimmune issue; however, the mechanism is not yet fully understood by scientists.

Type 2 diabetes, *on the other hand, is when the pancreas still produces insulin, but the body and its cells fail to respond to the insulin. This is called Insulin Resistance.*

It commonly affects the age groups of 30 or above, and develops over a long period of time - sometimes years. These patients can manage their diabetes with diet and exercise and in certain situations with natural hormones as well. The cause of this type of diabetes is usually due to poor dietary choices (excess carbohydrates) and the build-up of a lot of intra-abdominal fat (potbelly.) This is also directly related to excess estrogen within the body and a decline in testosterone and progesterone.

Conclusion: if weight gain is avoided then type 2 diabetes can be completely avoided.

Type 2 diabetes is much more common than Type 1.
Other causes of diabetes are:

1. Pregnancy aka gestational diabetes.
2. Acute and severe disease/ illness.
3. Medication (antibiotics and chemotherapy).
4. Pancreatitis.

Type 3 diabetes – Alzheimer's and neuro-degeneration of the brain – In 2005 Scientists at Brown Medical School[1] in the USA, had determined that

---

1 http://www.diabetesincontrol.com/index.php?option=com_content&view=article&id=2582. Accessed April 2012.

insulin is manufactured in the brain, and that lessened levels are linked to Alzheimer's disease.

> *"What we found is that insulin is not just produced in the pancreas, but also in the brain. And we discovered that insulin and its growth factors, which are necessary for the survival of brain cells, contribute to the progression of Alzheimer's,"* says senior author Suzanne M. de la Monte, a neuropathologist at Rhode Island Hospital and a professor of pathology at Brown Medical School.

This raises the possibility of a Type 3 *neuro*-degenerative diabetes, a form of "brain" diabetes. Its symptoms are called Alzheimer's and dementia.

Researchers and doctors discovered that insulin and insulin growth factor-1(IGF-1) were markedly reduced in the frontal cortex, hippocampus and hypothalamus - all regions that are disturbed by the advancement of Alzheimer's[2].

This book helps type 2 diabetics restore insulin sensitivity, and provides healthy support to brain tissue function and nerves. This means it will also helps type 3 diabetics.

This book cannot repair type 1 diabetes; however, following the dietary program will allow the Type 1 diabetic to require less insulin and, therefore, improve their quality of life[3].

Complications of diabetes will also be avoided.

Symptoms of Diabetes

Clearly diabetes is a sugar disease. Classic symptoms of diabetes are:

1. Loss of energy- very little sugar in the cells.
2. Excess urination- as the EXCESS sugar is excreted.
3. Thirst – because patients are urinating so much.
4. Recurring infections such as candidiasis - reduced immunity as sugar feeds bugs.

---

2   http://www.j-alz.com/press/2004/20040621.html. Accessed April 2012
3   Wolever TMS, Hamad S, Chiasson JL, Josse RG, Leiter LA, Rodger NW, et al. *Day-to-day consistency in amount and source of carbohydrate intake associated with improved glucose control in type 1 diabetes. J Am Coll Nutr.* 1999;18:242–247

5. Vision problems – eyes are very sensitive to sugar changes.
6. Kidney problems- aggravations from the excess sugar.

If you cut out all your sugars, including those that are hidden in 'bad' food choices, and start eating better food choices then your pancreas has a chance to heal. That's the start, and slowly you will see your body becoming healthier and all the symptoms of your diabetes will disappear.

Can you heal yourself from Diabetes type 2, with my guidance and your will power and determination?

Yes!

I know you can heal yourself from type 2 diabetes, and I have witnessed this in thousands of patients in my over 19 years of practice. It starts with the first ingredient in our diet, **sugar; also known as glucose, sucrose, carbohydrates and starches.**

Is there any modern scientific proof that going on a low calorie[4], low carbohydrate diet could possibly improve diabetes?

Yes. The evidence is strong that medical nutrition[5,6] is an effective and essential therapy in the management of diabetes and obesity whereby patients[7] can change their carbohydrate intake using a low calorie approach, use non-nutritive sweeteners, use Glycemic index control diets, and add more fiber to their diets, balance protein intake, and thereby reverse the risks of cardiovascular disease[8], and weight/obesity issues.

The most recent astonishing research has come out of the UK from a respected university.

---

4 Nielsen JV, Jonsson E, Nilsson AK. *Lasting improvement of hyperglycemia and body weight: Low-carbohydrate diet in type 2 diabetes* (A brief report). *Upsala J Med Sci.* 2005;109:179–184
5 Boden G, Sargrad K, Homko C, Mozzoli M, Stein TP. *Effect of a low-carbohydrate diet on appetite, blood glucose levels, and insulin resistance in obese patients with type 2 diabetes.* Ann Intern Med. 2005;142:403–411
6 Turner-McGrievy G, Barnard ND, Cohen J, Jenkins DJA, Gloede L, Green AA. *Changes in nutrient intake and dietary quality among participants with type 2 diabetes following a low-fat vegan diet or a conventional diabetes diet for 22 weeks. J Am Diet Assoc.* 2008;108:1636–1645
7 Nadeau J, Koski KG, Strychar I, Yale JF. *Teaching subjects with type 2 diabetes how to incorporate sugar choices into their daily meal plan promotes dietary compliance and does not deteriorated metabolic profile.* Diabetes Care. 2001;24:222–227
8 Jarvi AE, Karlstrom BE, Grandfeldt YE, Bjorck IE, Asp NGL, Vessby BOH. *Improved Glycemic control and lipid profile and normalized fibrinolytic activity on a low Glycemic index diet in type 2 diabetic patients.* Diabetes Care. 1999;22:10–18

The Newcastle University Study

A study has been conducted at Newcastle University, which has created a global controversy on how *few* calories are safe to eat. Most scientists believe that going below 1,000 calories per day can be risky to one's health and that was also what I had been taught. It was common practice to think that anything less than 1,000 calories required medical supervision on some level.

However, Roy Taylor, a professor at Newcastle University, monitored patients who'd had gastric bypass surgery[9]. Some of these patients also had Type 2 diabetes. After a couple of months of surgery these patients no longer had fat deposits on their organs (liver and pancreas) and therefore, no longer needed medication to control their blood sugar. Liver and pancreatic fat deposits found on MRI scans are a crucial sign of diabetes[10].

Taylor led a study to see if the sudden remission of Type 2 diabetes might be due to the extremely low calorie intake of post surgery patients and not due to the surgical removal of the patient's intestines. Some surgeons claimed that the removal of portions of the intestines, which produce certain substances, was responsible for the change in the patient's diabetes and the surgery was a cure for the disease. However, after gastric bypass surgery, patients could only eat very small amounts of food, which greatly limits their calorie intake. Taylor soon realized that the key to curing the diabetes was actually the reduced calories. Fasting caused the body to unplug the fat surrounding the pancreas[11].

In order to prove his theory, eleven people with type 2 diabetes took part in a study in which they cut their calories to 600 calories a day for two months. The study found that **seven of 11 obese individuals had a complete remission of their type 2 diabetes after being on the diet for eight weeks** (and losing an average of only 33 lbs). Surprisingly, this remission has lasted

---

9 Pories WJ, Caro JF, Flickinger EG, Meelheim HD, Swanson MS (1987) The control of diabetes mellitus (NIDDM) in the morbidly obese with the Greenville Gastric Bypass. Ann Surg 206:316–323
10 Lim EL, Hollingsworth KG, Aribisala BS, Chen MJ, Mathers JC, Taylor R. Reversal of type 2 diabetes: Normalisation of beta cell function in association with decreased pancreas and liver triacylglycerol. *Diabetologia* 2011, **54**(10), 2506-2514.
11 Lim EL, Hollingsworth KG, Aribisala BS, Chen MJ, Mathers JC, Taylor R. *Fasting Successfully Treats Early Diabetes Type 2*. Forschende Komplementaermedizin 2011, 18(6), 359-360. - http://www.ncl.ac.uk/biomedicine/research/groups/publication/180484

over 18 months so far, even though the average participant has regained almost seven lbs in that time frame.

Doctors from around the globe have claimed that this is not a diet, but 'starvation' and a very dangerous therapy for people with type 2 diabetes. However, one can argue that the process of healing is a "controlled fasting" technique. As patients lost weight (body fat) their diabetes improved greatly[12]. The MRI researchers have concluded that there is definitely a link between how fat someone is, and the levels of fat surrounding their liver and pancreas[13]. The MRI researchers concluded that fatty livers were closely related to overall weight gain, especially in central obesity.

Yet, the research from Prof. Roy Taylor showed that an extremely low-calorie diet prompted the body to remove the fat clogging the pancreas, which was preventing it from making insulin. This fat is most likely a major cause of type 2 diabetes.

After just one week on the low calorie diet, the pre-breakfast blood sugar levels of the study group had returned to normal, and MRI scans showed that the fat levels in the pancreas had started to disappear. This is good news for type 2 diabetics, and in effect it means that it has now been medically recognised that calorie restriction is an effective short-term strategy to reduce fasting blood sugars and lower body fat %.

Prof. Roy Taylor's ground-breaking study was recently revealed on a more international level in the Guardian Newspaper, UK [14] and his work was presented at the American Diabetes Association conference 2011.

Considering the incredible results, the lack of any invasive surgery or drugs required, and the short-term nature of the "treatment", it is hard to understand the outrage of the many doctors that have had to rethink their understanding of T2 Diabetes.

---

12   Lim EL, Hollingsworth KG, Aribisala BS, Chen MJ, Mathers JC, Taylor R. *Reversal of type 2 diabetes: Normalisation of beta cell function in association with decreased pancreas and liver triacylglycerol.* Diabetologia 2011, 54(10), 2506-2514.

13   E L Thomas, G Hamilton, N Patel, R O'Dwyer, C J Doré3, R D Goldin, J D Bell, S D Taylor-Robinson. Hepatic triglyceride content and its relation to body adiposity: a magnetic resonance imaging and proton magnetic resonance spectroscopy study- Int. *J. of Gastro/ Hepatology.* Gut 2005;54:122-127 doi:10.1136/gut.2003.036566

14   Sarah Boseley, *Low-calorie diet offers hope of cure for type 2 diabetes.* The Guardian, Friday 24 June 2011

There are some medical Doctors that puzzle at what has been discovered. Dr. Philip Schauer, professor of surgery and director of advanced laparoscopic & bariatric surgery at Cleveland Clinic, during a briefing at the American Diabetic Association conference said[15]:

"In my practice, I routinely see patients who have remission of their type 2 diabetes within days or hours of gastric bypass, but we don't know why this occurs,"

He continued by saying:

"Understanding how (bariatric) surgery has this effect has the potential to unlock new mechanisms of treating type 2 diabetes and, potentially, how to replicate the effect with less invasive procedures or even without surgery."

How to replicate the effect?

Throughout history, fasting and minimizing calorie intake has been considered an important part of health and well-being. Prof. Roy Taylor at Newcastle University has medically validated fasting to have a therapeutic effect on an ailing pancreas.

This is very similar to the calorie restriction effect of the modern "HCG diet" discovered in 1952 by British Medical trained physician, Dr Albert Simeons. We will cover this hot topic in Chapter One.

N.B.

Before embarking on any diabetic recovery program you must inform your physician to help guide you to the correct management of your medication. Detailed records of blood sugars and diet techniques must be taken so as to witness the changes that will occur. Your co-operation with your medical doctor,[16] together with good record keeping is essential, as it will be physiological proof that you are getting better.

---

15 http://medcitynews.com/2011/06/american-diabetes-association-conference-highlights-latest-research/
16 As your pancreas heals your MD will probably prescribe less and less medication for

Recommended regular tests are as follows:

- Blood glucose fasting
- Glucose tolerance test
- Uric acid test
- HBa1C
- Serum Insulin
- Urinalysis
- Cholesterol
- Blood pressure

Additional hormone testing:

- Thyroid panel – T3, T4, TSH
- Adrenal panel – DHEA and Cortisol
- Sex Hormones – testosterone, progesterone, E2

2. Yeast and Diabetes connection

Fungi are single-celled organisms, which can live in the earth, water and air. Most people know very little about the fungal kingdom. Fungi have lived on planet Earth for millions of years and surprisingly have changed very little over that time in terms of their DNA. These single celled organisms can only be seen under a microscope and yet when enough of them have grouped together they will form the molds on bread, or toadstools, on cow excreta and on trees - the list is endless.

The fungi themselves will eventually eat any creature that chooses to eat these fungi because the creature will die. Once death has taken over, the fungi will reduce the creature to its basic component parts and it is recycled from whence it came. However, fungi also have the ability to eat a living organism while it is still alive.

What people *must* know is that yeasts, mushrooms, mold, puffballs, mildews, and **fungi can hurt and kill humans and other mammals.** These fungi

---

Type 1 diabetics. If you are a Type 2 diabetic, you may have medication reduced until you can manage it with diet and exercise alone.

and their mycotoxins can be found in our food chain[17]. These mycotoxins can cause many diseases because they are composed of molecules that can block our human DNA function, damage our liver enzymes and "burn" our blood vessels[18], as observed by Prof. Costantini of retired head of the Centre for mycotoxins at the WHO.

It is therefore, very important that we manage our diet and remove our consumption of these fungi as much as possible. People also need to understand that fungi grow very slowly and it can take years before there are enough fungi in the body to create a super-infection, such as diabetes, obesity, heart disease, autoimmune diseases, some forms of MS, rheumatoid arthritis, strokes or cancer[19][20].

As I wrote in my first book '*The Hidden Cure,*' if the first Law[21] is followed, the result will be *less* chronic degenerative diseases. In my opinion, all chronic diseases should be investigated on a fungal sugar level, and the term chronic degenerative diseases should actually be reclassified as "chronic fungal degenerative diseases."

There are countless references that have associated fungi with weight gain and diabetes. Although fungi can break down or eat anything through their terrifyingly destructive mycotoxins, the key factor is that fungi like to eat simple foods such as carbohydrates.

Long-term, baker's and brewer's yeast can cause the body to start to feel the effects of the mycotoxins[22][23], which can lead to atherosclerosis, heart disease, diabetes and weight gain to name a few.

The antibiotic mycotoxin "cyclosporine", which is used routinely for

---

17   Sugar A. *A practical Guide to Medically Important Fungi and the Diseases they Cause*. Lippincot-Raven, Philadelphia,PA 1997
18   Costantini, AV, *Fungalbionics Series; Etiology and Prevention of Atherosclerosis*. Johann Freidrich Oberlin Verlag. Freiburg, Germany. 1998/99. Chp 1, pg 9-10
19   A A Stark. *Mutagenicity and Carcinogenicity of Mycotoxins: DNA Binding as a Possible Mode of Action* Annual Review of Microbiology Vol. 34: 235-262 (Volume publication date October 1980)
20   Wainwright, Milton. *Do fungi play a role in the aetiology of cancer?* Reviews in Medical Microbiology:January 2002 - Volume 13 - Issue 1 - pp 37-42
21   L. Maas B.Sc Ost, DI.Hom. *The Hidden Cure*. Wheatmark Pub. Chp. 5 pg 61. 2009
22   Costantini, AV, *Fungalbionics Series; Etiology and Prevention of Atherosclerosis*. Johann Freidrich Oberlin Verlag. Freiburg, Germany. 1998/99. Chp 9 pg 47-49
23   Ibid 43.Chp2 pg 28

transplant patients, will cause atherosclerosis and in some cases cancer[24]. Fungi and yeasts are routinely found in the food chain and are consumed regularly by unsuspecting humans.

Prof. Costantini, the retired head of the WHO Collaboration Centre for Mycotoxins in Foods, has carried out work that clearly shows fungi and their mycotoxins regularly colonize whole-wheat grains, corn kernels, peanuts, cashews, and dried coconut. Studies have shown that the insides of corn kernels and peanuts can be infested with fungus and that humans who eat these products are literally poisoning themselves without knowing it. Clear and concise advice is given by Costantini[25] in order to minimize the risks.

> *A person's dietary choices play the critical role in the causation or in the prevention of all the mycotoxin-related diseases, not only for adults but also for children. The selection of foods for children will determine the life expectancy and quality of health for these adults-to-be ... the diet must reduce the intake of mycotoxin-containing foods, not feed the fungi living within us, and decrease the toxicity of the mycotoxins, which do enter our bodies. Most important, is that the diet should exclude yeast-fermented foods. All other foods that are fresh and of high quality are acceptable.*

Even more recently an Italian surgical oncologist, Dr. Tullio Simoncini[26] has published a book titled '*Cancer is a Fungus*'. He is of the opinion that cancer is indeed a fungus that has its roots in Candida; he states that when he performs surgery on a cancer patient, he noted that the cancer was always white. Candida is also white in appearance. However, color is only one of the common threads. Histologically, the cancer cells have a metabolic similarity to Candida in that both need sugar to live. They produce a slew of mycotoxins, lactic acid and carbon dioxide. Nobel laureate Otto Heinrich Warburg stated[27]:

---

24 Ibid 44. Chp 7 pg 39
25 Ibid 44. Chp 2 Pg 18
26 Dr. T Simoncini, *Cancer is a Fungus*, Edizioni Lampis , Italy 2005
27 Warburg O (24 February 1956). "On the Origin of Cancer Cells". *Science* 123 (3191): 309–14.

"the prime cause of cancer is the replacement of the respiration of oxygen in normal body cells by a fermentation of sugar."

This hypothesis is known as the Warburg effect.

Warning about Leavened Bread

Bread and cereals cause obesity[28] [29] in children and is clinically correlated to atherosclerosis[30] in the older age groups. Bread is one of those yeasty food items that we eat all the time, during any season—for breakfast, lunch, snacks and dinner. Modern sliced bread contains very few nutrients due to the processing of the flour, which is why most bread has to be enriched[31] with vitamins. Enriched flour products tend to be higher on the Glycemic Index, quickly raising blood sugar levels.

Bread, having a high Glycemic Index, meaning it has a high sugar content, taxes the pancreas enormously, as it has to produce a rapid insulin response. A rapid insulin response is the body's way of controlling the sudden shift in blood sugar levels as a result of the bread's consumption.

If someone habitually eats junk food (wheat, sugar, flour, processed meat, artificial milkshakes, etc.), he or she causes swings in insulin, and as a result the pancreas will get 'tired.' If the junk food has yeast in it, or if that person is taking a course of antibiotics, then trouble will brew, literally.

Most consumers believe that bread is a solid staple, important to our diet, so it is worth taking a closer look at what we are really consuming and what the consequences are. A recent article[32] in *Ecologist* magazine stated that the yeast quantities in bread have increased over the last fifty years by 250%. Prior to World War II (WW2), the yeast level in the bread was approxi-

---

28 O'Connor M, Kiely D, Mulvihil M, Winters A, et al,: School Nutrition Survey. Ir Med J 86 (3); 89-91, 1993- http://www.ncbi.nlm.nih.gov/pubmed/8567245
29 Weker H. *Simple obesity in children. A study on the role of nutritional factors.* Med Wieku Rozwoj. 2006 Jan-Mar;10(1):3-191.- http://www.ncbi.nlm.nih.gov/pubmed/16733288
30 Cecil M. Burchfiel, Dwayne M. Reed, Ellen B. Marcus, Jack P. Strong, and Takuji Hayashi. *Association of Diabetes Mellitus with Coronary Atherosclerosis and Myocardial Lesions: An Autopsy Study from the Honolulu Heart Program.* Am. J. Epidemiol. (1993) 137(12): 1328-1340
31 Enriched Flour - http://en.wikipedia.org/wiki/Enriched_flour; accessed April 2012.
32 Jon Hughes & Pat Thomas, *BLT Sandwhich; The Big Lifestyle Trade-off,* Ecologist Magazine, 22nd September, 2006

mately 0.5% of the bread content. After WW2 the yeast levels in bread rose to 1.75%. The reason for this was the need for greater and faster amounts of quick-rising bread among the baby-boomer generation. As the population increased, massively, in Europe and North America so did the consumption of cheap, mass-produced bread.

At the same time in history, antibiotics had been discovered by Sir Alexander Fleming in 1928 [33] and were being used to treat patients, especially following WW2, when soldiers injured with shrapnel and bomb blasts needed them to cure bacterial infections. The children of this age came to think of antibiotics as a miracle. Very few people knew that antibiotics, such as Penicillin, were a refined form of fungal poison[34]. The only thing that can live in a fungal poison is another yeast or fungus.

It is precisely this generation and the ones thereafter that suffer from the most degenerative diseases such as Alzheimer's[35], cancer[36], heart disease[37] [38] [39] [40], obesity[41] and diabetes[42]. The repeated introduction of fermented foods, sugars, and beverages in an antibiotic-managed healthcare system has set up most of the degenerative diseases we see today. This is a crucial piece of evidence in the etiology of all chronic diseases effecting this baby-boom gen-

---

33   Diggins, F. *The true history of the discovery of penicillin by Alexander Fleming* Biomedical Scientist, March 2003, Insititute of Biomedical Sciences, London.
34   Penicillin, http://en.wikipedia.org/wiki/Penicillin
35   Alzheimer's Association. Alzheimer's Disease Facts and Figures 2008. - http://www.alz.org/national/documents/release_031808_2008_facts_and_figures.pdf 2008.
36   Baby-Boomer Cancer Epidemic forecast- University of South Florida, accessed April, 2012- http://www.research.usf.edu/spotlights.asp?id=5898
37   *Baby Boom to Elder Boom: Providing Health Care for an Aging Population.* Washington, D.C. Watson Wyatt Worldwide, 1996
38   *Sarah Worth, USF Health Communications,* Baby Boomers & Heart Disease, January 14, 2008 @ 11:53 am · Filed under Integrating USF Health
39   Sharon O'Brien, *Cost to Treat Heart Disease to Triple by 2030 as Baby Boomers Age, Prevention urgently needed to lower incidence and cost of heart disease.* About.com- http://seniorliving.about.com/od/hearthealth/a/Cost-To-Treat-Heart-Disease-To-Triple-By-2030-As-Baby-Boomers-Age.htm
40   Jason C. Kovacic, Pedro Moreno, Vladimir Hachinski, Elizabeth G. Nabel, and Valentin Fuster Circulation. *Contemporary Reviews in Cardiovascular Medicine, Cellular Senescence, Vascular Disease, and Aging*: Part 1 of a 2-Part Review.. 2011;123:1650-1660
41   J Gerontol B Psychol Sci Soc Sci (2009) 64B (3): 369-377.
42   Suzanne G. Leveille, PhD, Christina C. Wee, MD, MPH, and Lisa I. Iezzoni, MD, MSc, *Trends in Obesity and Arthritis Among Baby Boomers and Their Predecessors, 1971–2002,* American Journal of Public Health, September 2005, Vol 95, No. 9

eration. The BLT, The Lifestyle Tradeoff article[43] in the Ecologist magazine stated, "The increase in yeast is now being linked to a dramatic increase in yeast intolerance in the West."

'Curing type 2 diabetes in Seven Steps' aims to inform the reader of the benefits of going *yeast and wheat free*. Dr. Alessio Fasano, director of the University of Maryland Center for Celiac Research, stated that 2.5 to 3 million people in the USA have celiac disease. Unbeknownst to the general public, no more than 150,000 of them have been diagnosed, which in effect means that more than 2.3 million Americans are walking around with wheat and yeast allergies and don't know it. Not only is bread carrying more gluten and yeast[44], but so too is beer, beef, and bacon. So let's ask you some questions about yeast infections and wheat/ gluten allergies.

Are you sensitive to yeast / Candida?

Scroll down the list and see if you suffer from any of the following symptoms.

✓	✗	
		Skin rashes, Eczema/crustiness behind ears
		Itchy skin, hives
		Vaginal discharge
		Itchy, burning, painful sex
		Massive sugar cravings
		Cravings for alcohol
		Bad breath (halitosis)
		White coated tongue
		Recurring mouth ulcers
		Nail bed fungus
		Liver spots, skin fungus
		Headache, hangover

---

43 Jon Hughes & Pat Thomas, *BLT Sandwhich; The Big Lifestyle Trade-off*, Ecologist Magazine, 22nd September, 2006
44 Dr.LWilson.com: Food Sensitivities or Intolerance; Lawrence Wilson, M.D.; December 2010- http://www.drlwilson.com/articles/food_intolerance.htm

About Diabetes

✓	✗	
		Gas and bloating
		Painful urination
		White, flaky matter in the ear canal
		Acne
		Asthma, shortness of breath
		Gastric reflux/GERD/gastritis
		Cancer (Breast, Uterine, Prostate)
		Fibrocystic breast disease,
		Diabetes (Type 2)
		High cholesterol
		Gallstones
		Sinusitis
		Autoimmune diseases
		Depression/panic attacks
		Mental confusion
		Hypothyroidism and of course weight gain/obesity
		Arthritis, gout, and sub-acute gout
		PMS/mood swings due to serotonin fluctuations

Now count up how many "yes" answers you have and check your total against the table below:

0 to 2: Likely you are not yeast sensitive.

2 to 5: There is the possibility of a small issue, which is ever-increasing with each yes answer.

5 and over: Definite problem and recommended to cut out all yeast & wheat and gluten foods for at least three months.

Are you sensitive to wheat and gluten?

Take the quick test below by answering if you identify with any of these tendencies:

✔	✘	
		Difficulty gaining weight/ anorexic
		Difficulty losing weight
		Weight gain
		Tendency to get drunk easily
		Gassy after dairy products
		Have other food allergies
		Headaches/migraines
		Joint pain, swollen joints
		Hormone imbalances, mood swings
		Burpy, windy, gassy, farty
		Rashes on skin
		Bloated stomach after certain foods
		Cramping pains in the abdomen
		Crave sweets and candy
		Overeats carbs and sweets
		Overly sensitive/ cries easily
		Chronic fatigue
		Diabetes, sugar issues
		Anemia
		Candida / yeast infections
		Depression, low mood

Now count up how many "yes" answers you have and check your total against the table below:

0 to 4: Likely you are not gluten wheat sensitive.

5 to 10: There is the possibility of a small issue, which is increasing with each yes answer.

11 and over: Definite problem and recommended to cut out all wheat and gluten foods for at least 3 months.

Wheat and Gluten Sensitivities and Allergies

If you follow a gluten-free diet, you will be able to stabilize your blood sugar[45], gain improved liver function[46] and energy levels, have less migraines [47] and neuropathies, less eczema[48], reduce and remove cravings, have better bowel movements, get more sleep and also become slimmer. Some early research shows that a gluten free / casein free diet has wonderful benefits for autism[49].

Gluten sensitivity and Celiac disease are a known cause of scleroderma, rheumatoid[50], lupus and other auto-immune diseases. Even if other tests for gluten sensitivity and Celiac disease are negative or inconclusive, trial of a gluten-free and casein-free (GFCF) should be considered.

If you scored moderate to high numbers you should be gluten and wheat free for two-three months. This will allow your guts to heal from the allergic response to wheat within the gut lining.

Actually it's not quite an allergic response, it's more of an auto-immune response whereby the immune systems start to become corrupted and confused by the wheat/gluten proteins. The "friendly fire" starts to damage tissues, hence the link between auto-immune diseases, such as lupus and rheumatoid, and the chronic consumption of wheat based foods year in and year out.

Gluten intolerance is seriously under-diagnosed[51] [52]. Gluten sensitivity

---

45   Marc Y. Donath, Joachim Størling, Kathrin Maedler and Thomas Mandrup-Poulsen. Inflammatory mediators and islet ß-cell failure: a link between type 1 and type 2 diabetes. JOURNAL OF MOLECULAR MEDICINEVolume 81, Number 8 (2003), 455-470,
46   M.T. Bardella, L. Valenti, C. Pagliari, M. Peracchi, M. Farè, A.L. Fracanzani, S. Fargion, Searching for coeliac disease in patients with non-alcoholic fatty liver disease, Digestive and Liver Disease, Volume 36, Issue 5, May 2004, Pages 333-336, ISSN 1590-8658,
47   Grant EC (1979). "Food allergies and migraine". Lancet 1 (8123): 966–9.
48   Barnetson RS, Wright AL, Benton EC (1989). "IgE-mediated allergy in adults with severe atopic eczema". *Clin. Exp. Allergy* **19** (3): 321–5.
49   Elder JH (2008). "The gluten-free, casein-free diet in autism: an overview with clinical implications". Nutr Clin Pract 23 (6): 583–8.
50   Hvatum M, Kanerud L, Hällgren R, Brandtzaeg P (2006). "The gut–joint axis: cross reactive food antibodies in rheumatoid arthritis". Gut 55 (9): 1240–7.
51   Charlene Laino, *Celiac Disease Underdiagnosed?* WebMD Health News. May 20, 2008 - http://www.webmd.com/digestive-disorders/celiac-disease/news/20080520/celiac-disease-underdiagnosed
52   About Celiac Disease- http://www.gluten.net/learn/celiac-disease.aspx accessed April 2012

and intolerance appears to be more common in patients with insulin dependent diabetes[53]. Gluten can cause a wide range of symptoms from IBS to chronic allergies and even cancer and lupus. Not everyone is gluten intolerant, but it is advised that a two to three month period of removing gluten/wheat products from the diet will help everyone in so many ways.

As one removes wheat/gluten from the diet, the blood sugars will start to stabilize.

Gluten based foods include wheat, rye, oats, bulgur wheat, spelt, durum wheat, couscous, cream of wheat and semolina.

Starch based foods that are allowed in *small* amounts to replace wheat are quinoa, wild organic rice, millet, amaranth and buckwheat. When eating these grains make sure it is consumed with a good blood type protein as it will slow down the migration of carbohydrates into the blood.

Many gluten intolerant patients also have allergies to soy and dairy. These foods should also be avoided unless you knowingly understand that there is no allergy to these products.

Eggs are allowed. However, milk intolerance / lactose sensitivity is commonly associated with wheat and gluten. Readers should omit dairy for at least two weeks and then "test" the body with a piece of cheese or a glass of milk and see if there's a gas reaction or an allergy flare-up (i.e. eczema, sinus problems, headache or gastric reflux). In other words following a gluten-free and casein-free diet is very helpful.

N.B. It is seriously important to get the protein, carb and fat ratios correct when going gluten and wheat free. This information will be covered in the Chapter three/ Step three, which is all about metabolic type. Here you will be asked to work out the necessary ratios of your food by using your blood pressure levels, breath hold and taking the metabolic quiz in the book or on our website, but more on that later.

---

53   Michael J. Rensch, MD; John A. Merenich, MD; Michael Lieberman, PhD; Brian D. Long, BS, CRC; Dirk R. Davis, MD; and Peter R. McNally, DO. Gluten-Sensitive Enteropathy in Patients with Insulin-Dependent Diabetes Mellitus. Annals of Int Med.March 15, 1996, vol. 124 no. 6 564-567

3. The Diabetic Domino Effect

Sugar is an acid and acids can really hurt the body by upsetting its hormones and enzymes.

What is the Diabetic Dominoes Effect?

1. **Hyperglycemia** and insulin are acidic and very pro-inflammatory; this means that the two substances will scrape the insides of the cardiovascular system. To repair any damaged arteries and veins, the body uses cholesterol. This is one of the reasons why patients with insulin issues will also have progressively higher cholesterol levels.

2. **Inflammation** not only causes higher cholesterol but also a lot of free radicals. These free radicals can overpower our anti-oxidant reserve and this then causes damage to the DNA (genes), cells, organs and tissues. This in itself can cause cancer and heart disease. Uric acid builds up easily in a diabetic and is a major cause of arthritis and kidney disease. A low purine diet is essential to recover from this.

3. **Oxygen** is normally carried by the red blood cells, but these red blood cells change and now preferentially remove the oxygen and carry the glucose instead. This lowers the body's oxygenation level. Low oxygen leads to thicker blood and further disease; this usually manifests as hypertension, low energy levels, arthritis, diabetic blindness, the development of gangrenous tissue and eventually to limb amputation.

4. **Thicker blood-** as the blood gets thicker the brain tries to remedy the situation by making the host thirsty and of course the patient drinks more water in order to dilute the blood. Increased water consumption causes the body to urinate more and this causes the loss of precious alkalizing minerals.

5. **Hypertension-** as the blood becomes thicker, the heart has to pump the blood around with increased pressure and this is detrimental to the heart, kidneys and brain.

6. **Weight gain and Obesity-** it's now well established that the greater the insulin resistance, the greater the development of fat cells. These

two are inextricably linked. To lose weight one must control the flow of carbohydrates going into the body. You can do this by choosing low GI foods.

7. **Death** of the pancreatic tissues (Islets of Langerhans) and the diagnosis of Type 1 diabetes. This condition requires vigilant insulin management with a good diet and exercise program.

4. How to heal the sugar function of the pancreas

The pancreas is a very important gland in that it both secretes hormones into the blood and excretes hormones and enzymes into the digestive system. A group of very specialized cells (approximately 1 million) called the Islets of Langerhans are responsible for making insulin.

The cause of T2 diabetes is diet and obesity, and not a lack of a drug. The issue is the amount of glucose in the diet and how it affects insulin *resistance*. Bad food choices create insulin resistance and in order to fix it one must start to make proper food choices. Both the carbohydrate choice and the portion play a significant role in determining postprandial insulin responses.

When you eat some food your body will take the carbohydrate and break it down into smaller molecules called glucose. Insulin is needed by the cells of the body to allow the glucose to get into the cells.

Insulin is like a "Stage Pass" that allows the glucose to "enter" the cell. Insulin's main job is to store sugar, which will eventually turn into fat.

By reducing the glucose load in the body at each meal (using a low GI diet) one can reduce the amount of insulin secreted and allow the pancreas to recover, this in turn allows for weight loss and reduction in blood pressure.

How do you fix it naturally?

1. Have your diabetes tests performed and evaluated by your MD, DO, ND, DC or registered nurse (RN).
2. Start a *gentle* exercise routine with your personal trainer (30 mins - 45 mins per day, 3 -5 x per week).
3. Start eating a low Glycemic Index diet. **ALLWAYS** have carbs and pro-

About Diabetes

tein together. *Never eat carb by itself.* Think fruit and nut, e.g. apples and almonds or vegetables and meat/ fish/ fowl.

4. Eat proteins regularly based on blood type.
5. Eat good fats like fish oils, flax and olive oil.
6. Eat a diet full of the anti-oxidants found in vegetables.
7. Increase your fiber to help regulate the flow of carbohydrates into the blood.
8. Eat cinnamon daily.
9. Eat garlic daily.
10. Eat regularly, like every 3 hours.
11. Have regular meals **ON TIME**.
12. Have protein snacks in between meals.
13. Exercise regularly- research has shown that exercise is excellent at improving insulin sensitivity. Patients can double their insulin efficiency within six months.
14. Reduce your stress levels through meditation, yoga, prayer and silent contemplation.
15. Use positive visualization - this helps to reduce anxiety by guiding your mind to create positive outcomes for the future, instead of negative thoughts about the future.

What supplements will improve my Pancreas?

One product that I have found to be outstanding is a powdered shake called UltraGlycemX [54]. It contains all the necessary ingredients to help Type 2 diabetics regain pancreatic control. UltraGlycemx has been clinically tested and is extremely convenient. UltraGlycemx testing shows that it parallels other lifestyle data. Lifestyle changes were cited in the New England journal of Medicine, Feb 7 2002[55].

---

54 Dan Lukaczer, ND, Barbara Schiltz, RN, MS, CN,, *Determination of the Glycemic Index for UltraGlycemXTM Medical Food*. Research Report Number 106 – Functional Medicine Research Center, Gig Harbor, WA 98335 July 7, 2000

55 Diabetes Prevention program Research Group. N Engl J Med 2002; 346:393-403. Feb 7 2002

"Lifestyle changes and treatment with Metformin both reduced the incidence of diabetes in persons at high risk. The lifestyle intervention was more effective than Metformin."

UltraGlycemX has proved to be effective in Type 2 diabetes in over 37 clinical trials. It improves insulin sensitivity, pancreatic function and encourages weight loss through proper cholesterol and fat metabolism when combined with 2-3 grams of omega oils per day.

Other supplements found to be scientifically helpful are:
- Co Q10
- Chromium
- Magnesium
- Alpha-lipoic acid
- Goats Rue Extract
- Gymnema
- Omega 3,6,9 (2-3g/day)

All of the supplements and hormones listed will help to reduce inflammation, improve oxygenation of the tissues, and stabilize blood sugar. Below are descriptions of the outstanding supplements.

CoQ10 – is a powerful anti-oxidant. It is a fat soluble nutrient that favours the recovery of the Beta cells of the pancreas, those cells responsible for making insulin. CoQ10 is also helpful in reducing the symptoms of angina, congestive heart issues[56] and heart valve dysfunctions, and also helps to lower blood pressure[57,58]. These are all related to CoQ10 deficiencies and are somehow linked to T2 diabetes. CoQ10 is a natural anti-fungal substance. Suggested doses per day range from 60-300mg depending on the amount of pancreatic and cardiac support needed.

---

56 Dhanasekaran M, Ren J. The emerging role of coenzyme Q-10 in aging, neurodegeneration, cardiovascular disease, cancer and diabetes mellitus. *Curr Neurovasc Res.* 2005;2(5):447-59.
57 Hodgson JM, Watts GF, Playford DA, et al. Coenzyme Q(10) improves blood pressure and glycaemic control: a controlled trial in subjects with type 2 diabetes. *Eur J Clin Nutr.* 2002;56:1137-1142.
58 Rosenfeldt F, Hilton D, Pepe S, Krum H. *Systematic review of effect of coenzyme Q10 in physical exercise, hypertension and heart failure.* Biofactors. 2003;18(1-4):91-100.

Chromium – Lowers HbA1C levels, encourages weight loss and prevents insulin resistance. Many obese and diabetic patients are chromium deficient thereby increasing insulin activity. Chromium is depleted when individuals eat a refined carbohydrate diet. Chromium is absolutely essential to normal glucose metabolism and it is fundamental in shunting glucose into the cell for storage and energy production. Combined with Alpha-Lipoic acid they make for a formidable combination in the fight against fat and diabetes. Patients with diabetes should have a minimum daily amount of 500mcg; however, once again, keen observation of blood glucose levels need to be maintained as this product works effectively. Guidance of a physician is always advised when drug management is concerned with diabetics. One 1997 study found that 1,000 mcg of chromium picolinate daily completely corrected Type II diabetes[59].

Magnesium- This alkalizing mineral helps to improve insulin function within the body[60][61][62], reduces stress responses, lowers blood pressure[63] and helps with good bowel movements (parasympathetic activity). It is absolutely essential to correct magnesium levels in the T2 Diabetic human body[64]. Failure to do so will impede any Diabesity recovery program. When magnesium is lacking, the body will cause the insulin levels to rise, which will in turn increase the blood sugar levels[65].

As a mineral supplement Magnesium is used in the body in hundreds of chemical reactions (more than 300) and is particularly used in the production of ATP, the body's source of energy. Plants are green because of magne-

---

59   R A Anderson, N Cheng, N A Bryden, M M Polansky, N Cheng, J Chi and J Feng. *Elevated intakes of supplemental chromium improve glucose and insulin variables in individuals with type 2 diabetes.* Diabetes November 1997 vol. 46 no. 11 1786-1791
60   Tosiello L. Hypomagnesemia and diabetes mellitus. A review of clinical implications. Arch Intern Med 1996;156:1143-8.
61   Paolisso G, Scheen A, D'Onofrio F, Lefebvre P. Magnesium and glucose homeostasis. Diabetologia 1990;33:511-4
62   Kobrin SM and Goldfarb S. Magnesium Deficiency. Semin Nephrol 1990;10:525-35.
63   Ascherio A, Rimm EB, Giovannucci EL, Colditz GA, Rosner B, Willett WC, Sacks FM, Stampfer MJ. A prospective study of nutritional factors and hypertension among US men. Circulation 1992;86:1475-84.
64   Fernando Guerrero-Romero, Martha Rodríguez-Morán, Complementary Therapies for Diabetes: The Case for Chromium, Magnesium, and Antioxidants, Archives of Medical Research, Volume 36, Issue 3, May–June 2005, Pages 250-257, ISSN 0188-4409, 10.1016/j.arcmed.2005.01.004
65   American Diabetes Association. Nutrition recommendations and principles for people with diabetes mellitus. Diabetes Care 1999;22:542-5.

sium, which is the essential component of chlorophyll. Cocoa, vegetables, nuts and spices are good sources of magnesium.

Alpha-Lipoic Acid - A powerful anti-oxidant that lowers insulin and blood glucose levels, and also helps to burn fat within the cells. It aids mitochondrial function and helps to create more energy. If glucose is used by the cell's mitochondria in an orderly and consistent fashion then energy is increased. Alpha-lipoic acid prevents the buildup of free radicals within the heart and blood vessels[66]. Moderate to high doses show great changes in blood glucose levels[67] so you must monitor and evaluate the effects. Doses of between 250-600 mg are normal. High doses of 1000 -1500mg need the careful watch of a physician.

L-Carnitine – increases insulin sensitivity[68] and glucose storage[69] within the cell, improves HbA1C levels[70]; helps to prevent cardiomyopathy, a condition commonly seen in diabetics and obese patients. Doses range from 500 - 1000mg per day.

Goat's Rue Extract - this herb is native to Europe and Britain[71] and has been used to control blood sugar due to a specific compound called guanidine. Guanidine has a specific effect for resensitising insulin within the body. Studies on Goat's Rue extract gave rise to the pharmaceutical Metformin[72] (Glucophage). This is a major anti-diabetic biguanide, which clinically demonstrates a blood sugar lowering capacity, helps to reduce body fat, improves lipid profiles and increases lifespan.

Goat's rue extract is thought to work by improving the membrane sen-

---

66   Peter Kempler, Review: Autonomic neuropathy: a marker of cardiovascular risk Department of Medicine, Semmelweis University, British Journal of Diabetes & Vascular Disease March 2003 vol. 3 no. 2 84-90
67   Diabetes und Stoffwechsel, 1996, vol. 5, Supp 3; American Journal of Clinical Nutrition, 1993, vol. 57; 1994, vol. 60
68   Mingrone G. Carnitine in type 2 diabetes. Ann NY Acad Sci 2004;1033:99-107
69   De Gaetano A, Mingrone G, Castagneto M, Calvani M. Carnitine increases glucose disposal in humans. J Am Coll Nutr 1999;18:289-95
70   Mingrone G, Greco AV, Capristo E, Benedetti G, Giancaterini A, De Gaetano A, Gasbarrini G. L-carnitine improves glucose disposal in type 2 diabetic patients. J Am Coll Nutr 1999;77-82
71   Witters, L. A. (2001). "The blooming of the French lilac". *Journal of Clinical Investigation* 2001, Oct 15, 108 (8): 1105–7
72   Bailey CJ, Day, C. (2004). "Metformin: its botanical background". *Practical Diabetes Int* 21 (3): 115–117

sitivity of cells to insulin's signal. As we age or overload our body with excess sugars, our cell membranes become less sensitive to the insulin signals. Goats rue extract rejuvenates the cell membranes to the chemical insulin signal, thereby allowing uptake of sugars by the cell and lowering the levels of blood sugar. Goat's Rue extract does not trigger hypoglycemia and is also known to prevent blood clots, diabetic retinopathy as well as protects the kidneys.

Gymnema Sylvestre - otherwise known as a 'sugar destroyer', this is an Ayurvedic herbal medicine used for thousands of years in India to treat hyperglycemia[73][74]. Gymnema has also been used to treat sugar cravings by altering the taste sensation of sugar in the tongue receptors. Gymnema, like Goat's Rue extract, does not induce the hypoglycemia – i.e. the hypoglycemia reactions that are sometimes seen with the use of insulin or the sulphonylurea drugs used to treat diabetes.

Gymnema can also be used to treat weight issues and obesity[75]. Gymnema is a very safe herb to take to help control type 2 diabetes and aids in the recovery of insulin sensitivity in the body as it promotes the recovery of the pancreas.

5. The Omega Oils

Oil supplements are very beneficial to help fix the pancreas[76][77] function and helps to lower triglycerides and other fats[78]. The best oils are:

---

[73] K. Baskaran, B.Kizar Ahamath, K.Radha Shanmugasundaram, E.R.B. Shanmugasundaram, Antidiabetic effect of a leaf extract from Gymnema sylvestre in non-insulin-dependent diabetes mellitus patients, Journal of Ethnopharmacology, Volume 30, Issue 3, October 1990, Pages 295-305,
[74] E.R.B. Shanmugasundaram, G. Rajeswari, K. Baskaran, B.R.Rajesh Kumar, K.Radha Shanmugasundaram, B.Kizar Ahmath, Use of Gymnema sylvestre leaf extract in the control of blood glucose in insulin-dependent diabetes mellitus, Journal of Ethnopharmacology, Volume 30, Issue 3, October 1990, Pages 281-294
[75] Preuss, H. G., Bagchi, D., Bagchi, M., Rao, C. V. S., Dey, D. K. and Satyanarayana, S. (2004), Effects of a natural extract of (-)-hydroxycitric acid (HCA-SX) and a combination of HCA-SX plus niacin-bound chromium and *Gymnema sylvestre* extract on weight loss. Diabetes, Obesity and Metabolism, 6: 171–180
[76] Cylla E Friedberg, MD, Martien J F M Janssen, PHD, MD, Robert J Heine, PHD, MD and Diederick E Grobbee, PHD, MD. Fish Oil and Glycemic Control in Diabetes: A meta-analysis, Diabetes Care April 1998 vol. 21 no. 4 494-500
[77] Riediger ND, Othman RA, Suh M, Moghadasian MH. A systemic review of the roles of n-3 fatty acids in health and disease. *J Am Diet Assoc.* 2009 Apr;109(4):668-79.
[78] Popp-Snijders C, Schouten JA, Heine RJ, van der Meer J, van der Veen EA, Dietary

Olive oil, Omega 9

This is one of the most remarkable oils in the history of mankind. No other oil can perform as well as Olive oil in terms of improving human health[79]. Olive oil was used as a fuel, food and as a medicinal remedy that could be absorbed directly by the skin. Olive oil is an Omega 9 oil; our bodies are made from it together with Omega 3's and 6's. Olive oil is referenced over 200 times in the Bible and is always associated with wellness and purity.

Olive oil comes from olive trees. All across the Middle East olive trees grow. These trees are known for their longevity and those humans, particularly Mediterranean Europeans[80] who consume it regularly will swear by it as life extending[81] oil. Europeans generally have less heart disease and less hypertension than their American counterparts.

Olive oil can perform all these wonderful medical functions:

- Conditions the hair and skin naturally.
- Fantastic for treating wounds together with Aloes and Myrrh.
- Relieves constipation.
- Gives energy.
- Balances blood pressure.

---

supplementation of omega-3 polyunsaturated fatty acids improves insulin sensitivity in non-insulin-dependent diabetes., Diabetes research (Edinburgh, Scotland) [1987, 4(3):141-7]

79   J. López-Miranda, F. Pérez-Jiménez, E. Ros, R. De Caterina, L. Badimón, M.I. Covas, E. Escrich, J.M. Ordovás, F. Soriguer, R. Abiá, C. Alarcón de la Lastra, M. Battino, D. Corella, J. Chamorro-Quirós, J. Delgado-Lista, D. Giugliano, K. Esposito, R. Estruch, J.M. Fernandez-Real, J.J. Gaforio, C. La Vecchia, D. Lairon, F. López-Segura, P. Mata, J.A. Menéndez, F.J. Muriana, J. Osada, D.B. Panagiotakos, J.A. Paniagua, P. Pérez-Martinez, J. Perona, M.A. Peinado, M. Pineda-Priego, H.E. Poulsen, J.L. Quiles, M.C. Ramírez-Tortosa, J. Ruano, L. Serra-Majem, R. Solá, M. Solanas, V. Solfrizzi, R. de la Torre-Fornell, A. Trichopoulou, M. Uceda, J.M. Villalba-Montoro, J.R. Villar-Ortiz, F. Visioli, N. Yiannakouris, Olive oil and health: Summary of the II international conference on olive oil and health consensus report, Jaén and Córdoba (Spain) 2008, Nutrition, Metabolism and Cardiovascular Diseases, Volume 20, Issue 4, May 2010, Pages 284-294

80   Esposito K, Marfella R, Ciotola M, et al. Effect of a mediterranean-style diet on endothelial dysfunction and
markers of vascular inflammation in the metabolic syndromea randomized trial. JAMA. 2004;292(12):1440-1446.

81   Knoops KB, de Groot LM, Kromhout D, et al. Mediterranean diet, lifestyle factors, and 10-year mortality in elderly
european men and womenthe hale project. JAMA. 2004;292(12):1433-1439

- Helps with osteoarthritis.
- Protects the heart and blood vessels.
- Reduces the bad cholesterol, LDL.
- Increases the good cholesterol, HDL.
- Prevents blood platelets from Rouleaux or sticking together.
- Protects the body from cancer by making the physiology catabolic, thereby allowing the body to break down pre-malignant or cancer cells.
- Encourages proper bile flow and Liver and Gall Bladder function.
- Relieves gastric reflux by soothing irritated stomach tissue.

Fish Oils, Omega 3

These oils from fish are, like olive oil, very protective to the heart and cardiovascular system[82]. It is a well-known fact, that those people who consume regular doses of fish oils have less heart disease and strokes. Those patients also report having improved memory and brain function as the brain and nerves are made from these oils.

In many fish oils there is also small amounts of Vitamin A and D and these can help the immune system ward off viruses and improve eyesight and bone density.

The oil actually protects the lining of the vascular system by making it very smooth[83] and therefore there is less friction in the flow of blood through the blood vessels; this oil is therefore called an endo-protectant. 'endo' means inside and 'protectant' means it shields the vessels. This oil works by reducing inflammation[84]. Inflammatory substances such as cytokines, prostaglandins, leukotrienes and thromboxanes cause the body to become irritated. This irritation can cause inflammatory diseases such as arthritis, asthma, irritable

---

[82] Alexander Leaf, MD; Jing X. Kang, MD, PhD; Yong-Fu Xiao, MD, PhD; George E. Billman, PhD. *Clinical Prevention of Sudden Cardiac Death by n-3 Polyunsaturated Fatty Acids and Mechanism of Prevention of Arrhythmias by n-3 Fish Oils.* Circulation. 2003; 107: 2646-2652

[83] HA Lehr, C Hubner, B Finckh, D Nolte, U Beisiegel, A Kohlschutter and K Messmer. *Dietary fish oil reduces leukocyte/endothelium interaction following systemic administration of oxidatively modified low density lipoprotein.* Circulation. 1991; 84: 1725-1731

[84] J E Kinsella, B Lokesh, and R A Stone. *Dietary n-3 polyunsaturated fatty acids and amelioration of cardiovascular disease: possible mechanisms.* Am J Clin Nutr July 1990 52: 1-28

bowel syndrome, eczema and psoriasis, diverticulitis and colitis. Fish oils prevent the build of inflammatory cytokines[85].

Fish Oils can:

- Reduce blood clots and therefore the risk of stroke[86] as it thins the blood naturally[87].
- Reduce blood pressure[88].
- Improve osteo-arthritis[89] [90].
- Improve asthma, bronchitis and other lung conditions[91].
- Improve diabetes by allowing the cells to absorb more glucose and thereby reduces blood sugar[92].
- Improve eczema both internally and externally on the skin[93].
- Help with multiple sclerosis[94] (hardening of the nerves).

---

85   Calder PC. n-3 Polyunsaturated Fatty Acids and Cytokine Production in Health and Disease, *Ann Nutr Metab 1997;41:203–234*
86   Kirpal S. Sidhu, Health benefits and potential risks related to consumption of fish or fish oil, Regulatory Toxicology and Pharmacology, Volume 38, Issue 3, December 2003, Pages 336-344,
87   A.Leaf MD. Cardiovascular effects of fish oils. Beyond the platelet. Circulation 1990, 82:624-628
88   Howard R. Knapp, M.D., Ph.D., and Garret A. FitzGerald, M.D. The Antihypertensive Effects of Fish Oil. N Engl J Med 1989; 320:1037-1043April 20, 1989
89   Vijitha De Silva, Ashraf El-Metwally, Edzard Ernst George Lewith and Gary J. Macfarlane. Evidence for the efficacy of complementary and alternative medicines in the management of osteoarthritis: a systematic review. Rheumatology (2011) 50 (5): 911-920.
90   T Stammers, B Sibbald, P Freeling, Efficacy of cod liver oil as an adjunct to non-steroidal anti-inflammatory drug treatment in the management of osteoarthritis in general practice. Ann Rheum Dis 1992;51:128-129
91   T Nagakura, S Matsuda, K Shichijyo, H Sugimoto and K Hata. Dietary supplementation with fish oil rich in omega-3 polyunsaturated fatty acids in children with bronchial asthma. ERJ November 1, 2000 vol. 16 no. 5 861-865
92   P Fasching, K Ratheiser, W Waldhäusl, M Rohac, W Osterrode, P Nowotny and H Vierhapper. Metabolic effects of fish-oil supplementation in patients with impaired glucose tolerance. Diabetes May 1991 vol. 40 no. 5 583-589
93   Craig C Miller, Wilson Tang, Vincent A Ziboh and Mark P Fletcher. Dietary Supplementation with Ethyl Ester Concentrates of Fish Oil (n-3) and Borage Oil (n-6) Polyunsaturated Fatty Acids Induces Epidermal Generation of Local Putative Anti-Inflammatory Metabolites. *Journal of Investigative Dermatology* (1991) 96, 98–103
94   Kenneth K. Carroll, Biological effects of fish oils in relation to chronic diseases. LIPIDS, Volume 21, Number 12 (1986), 731-732

- Help with athero-sclerosis (hardening of the arteries) by reducing cholesterol[95].
- Relieve the pain of colitis[96] (inflammation of the colon).
- Herring, Sardines, Mackerel, Tuna, and Salmon are all great sources of these fish oils.
- If a patient is intolerant of the "fish" oils then nature has provided a source of Omega 3's from the land in the form of Linseed or Flax seed oils and Hemp oil.

6. Natural Hormone Therapy

The natural hormones Pregnenolone[97], DHEA[98,99,100], Estrogen[101], Progesterone and Testosterone[102,103], and the HCG[104] diet all have beneficial effects in reversing diabetes (T2), lowering weight / obesity[105], lowering cho-

---

95 Ibid 104.
96 Maintenance of Remission in Inflammatory Bowel Disease Using Omega-3 Fatty Acids (Fish Oil): A Systematic Review and Meta-Analyses. *Nutr Clin Pract* 2011;26:2 202-203
97 Andreen L, Sundstrom-Poromaa I, Bixo M, Nyberg S, Backstrom T. Allopregnanolone concentration and mood--a bimodal association in postmenopausal women treated with oral progesterone. Psychopharmacology (Berl). 2006 Aug;187(2):209-21.
98 Hiroaki Kawano, Hirofumi Yasue, Akira Kitagawa, Nobutaka Hirai, Toshiaki Yoshida, Hirofumi Soejima, Shinzo Miyamoto, Masahiro Nakano and Hisao Ogawa. The Journal of Clinical Endocrinology & Metabolism , DHEA Supplementation Improves Endothelial Function and Insulin Sensitivity in Men, July 1, 2003 vol. 88 no. 7 3190-3195
99 Enomoto M, Adachi H, Fukami A, Furuki K, Satoh A, Otsuka M, Kimagae S, Nanjo Y, Shigetoh Y, Imaizumi T. Serum dehydroepiandrosterone sulfate levels predict longevity in men: 27-year follow-up study in a community-based cohort (Tanushimaru study). *J Am Geriatr Soc* 2008;56:994-8
100 Weiss EP, Villareal DT, Fontana L, Han DH, Holloszy JO. Dehydroepiandrosterone (DHEA) replacement decreases insulin resistance and lowers inflammatory cytokines in aging humans. *Aging (Albany NY)* 2011 May 10.
101 Katerina Saltiki, Maria Alevizaki. Coronary heart disease in postmenopausal women; the role of endogenous estrogens and their receptors. Athens University School of Medicine. HORMONES 2007, 6(1):9-24
102 D Kapoor, E Goodwin, K S Channer and T H Jones. Testosterone replacement therapy improves insulin resistance, glycaemic control, visceral adiposity and hypercholesterolaemia in hypogonadal men with type 2 diabetes Eur J Endocrinol June 1, 2006 154 899-906
103 Mårin P, Holmäng S, Jönsson L, Sjöström L, Kvist H, Holm G, Lindstedt G, Björntorp P. The effects of testosterone treatment on body composition and metabolism in middle-aged obese men. International journal of obesity and related metabolic disorders : journal of the International Association for the Study of Obesity [1992, 16(12):991- 997
104 Clegg DJ, Brown LM, Woods SC, Benoit SC, 2006 Gonadal hormones determine sensitivity to central leptin and insulin. Diabetes 55: 978-987
105 Shoelson SE,Herrero L, Naaz A. Obesity, inflammation, and insulin resistance. *Gastro-*

lesterol[106] and improving eyesight[107], heart disease[108] and libido[109][110]. Hormones work really well when given under the correct medical supervision and dose.

However, I only encourage my patients to use *bio-identical hormones* at my clinic and NEVER synthetic ones due to the associated negative side effects of them; and so I give you, the reader, the same advice as my patients. Bio-identical hormones are much safer than synthetic hormones, especially if the method of delivery is a cream or liposomal liquid. The advantage of this is that they bypass the liver, which would normally break them down quite quickly.

It is not so well known amongst medical practitioners that low dose natural hormone replacement can help to reverse diabetes. We will cover this area in the third lesson – Step 3 / chapter 3.

I would strongly advise my patients to get accurate comprehensive blood hormone panels and have the test results properly assessed by a competent physician trained in natural hormone replacement therapy. Use only optimal ranges when assessing the need for natural hormone replacement therapy.

Reassessing the hormones every three months is a good feedback technique until the hormones are all within balance.

7. The HCG Diet

The HCG diet is based on the work of Dr. Albert Simeons (1900–1970), a British trained Medical Doctor who recommended an ultra-low calorie diet (minimal carbohydrates) together with small doses of HCG, a

---

enterology 2007;132:2169-80.
106 Dzugan SA, Smith RA. Broad spectrum restoration in natural steroid hormones as possible treatment for hypercholesterolemia. Bull Urg Rec Med. 2002;3:278-84.
107 Tamer C, Oksuz H, Sogut S. Serum dehydroepiandrosterone sulphate level in age-related macular degeneration. Am J Ophthalmol. 2007 Feb;143(2):212-6.
108 Thijs L, Fagard R, Forette F, Nawrot T, Staessen JA. Are low dehydroepiandrosterone sulphate levels predictive for cardiovascular diseases? A review of prospective and retrospective studies. Acta Cardiol. 2003 Oct;58(5):403-10.
109 Decreased Free Testosterone and Dehydroepiandrosterone-sulfate (DHEA-S) Levels in Women with Decreased Libido, A. T. Guay, Jerilynn Jacobson Journal of Sex & Marital Therapy Vol. 28, Iss. sup1, 2002
110 Thomas G. Travison, John E. Morley, Andre B. Araujo, Amy B. O'Donnell and John B. McKinlay, The Relationship between Libido and Testosterone Levels in Aging MenThe Journal of Clinical Endocrinology & Metabolism July 1, 2006 vol. 91 no. 7 2509-2513

hormone produced during pregnancy that stimulates the body to produce more testosterone in males and more progesterone in females.

The action of HCG is virtually identical to that of pituitary LH, although HCG appears to have a small degree of FSH activity as well. It stimulates production of gonadal steroid hormones by stimulating the interstitial cells (Leydig cells) of the testis to produce androgens and the corpus luteum of the ovary to produce progesterone[111].

The increased production of those hormones in conjunction with a very low calorie diet causes the body to burn off a lot of fat very rapidly[112]. Proponents of the HCG diet maintains structural fat and only burns off abnormal fat reserves so that there is no 'skin sag', and observations in patients seem to hold true.

The program usually lasts 26-43 days at the most, and then the patient has to move onto a maintenance phase for six weeks to help reprogram the brain to the new 'set' weight point. This was important, as Dr Simeons believed that the 'chip set' within the brain would remember to have the right level of metabolism for the person's weight.

Be sure to check with your doctor if you have any concerns with your diabetes and HCG diet programs. However, this is what, the discoverer of the HCG diet, had to say on the subject of HCG and diabetes:

> *"In an obese patient suffering from a fairly advanced case of stable diabetes [Type II diabetes] of many years duration in which the blood sugar may range from 3-400 mg%, it is often possible to stop all anti-diabetic medication after the first few days of treatment [with HCG]. The blood sugar continues to drop from day to day and often reaches normal values in 2-3 weeks. As in pregnancy, this phenomenon is not observed in [Type I diabetes], and as some cases that are predominantly stable may have small Type 1 tendencies in their clinical makeup, all obese diabetics have to be kept under a very careful and expert watch.*

---

111   Drugs.com, Pregnyl HCG, http://www.drugs.com/pro/pregnyl.html; accessed April 2012
112   Dr. Daniel Belluscio, Dr. Leonor Ripamonte, Dr. Marcelo Wolansky. UTILITY OF AN ORAL PRESENTATION OF hCG (human Choriogonadotropin) FOR THE MANAGEMENT OF OBESITY. A DOUBLE-BLIND STUDY- *1994-2007-* http://oralhcg.com/english/hCG_Double_Blind_Study.pdf

> *Type 1 diabetes occurs, primarily, due to the inability of the pancreas to produce sufficient insulin, while in the type 2 diabetic, diencephalon regulations seem to be of greater importance. That is possibly the reason why Type 2 diabetes responds so well to the HCG method of treating obesity, whereas the Type 1 does not.*
>
> *Obese patients are generally suffering from the T 2, but a stable type may gradually change into a Type 1 diabetic, which is usually associated with a loss of weight. Thus, when an obese diabetic finds that he is losing weight without diet or treatment, he should at once have his diabetes expertly attended to. There is some evidence to suggest that the change from Type 2 to Type 1 (Insulin dependent) is more liable to occur in patients who are taking insulin for their stable diabetes."* Dr. Albert Simeons

As you well know from previous examples of diabetic remission (the Newcastle study and the Calorie Restricted diets), the HCG diet is also low in calories. To be precise the calorie intake is only 500 – 800 calories; however, the HCG hormones boost the progesterone and testosterone levels[113] so that the extra calories needed by the body come from the metabolism of their own fat reserves approximately 1,500-3,000 calories in fat burn/ day.

Patients really can lose up to a 1lb or more of fat per day. I have professionally witnessed this at my clinic.

FYI: 3,000 calories = 1 lb of fat

Many people are successfully using the HCG diet plan in order to drop extra pounds rapidly. While every individual is unique and he or she may or may not face health challenges, the HCG dieting plan is proving quite beneficial for users with a variety of pre-existing health conditions.

Even some individuals with diabetes are looking for positive ways to manage their weight, and the HCG diet can be used in order to achieve weight loss success even if a person is a diabetic.

The type of diabetes a person has will determine if the HCG dieting plan is a good dieting plan for the individual. Some people endure a form of diabetes identified as Stable Diabetes or Type 2 Diabetes. People with this form of diabetes can definitely benefit from the HCG dieting plan. However,

---

113 Drugs.com, Pregnyl HCG, http://www.drugs.com/pro/pregnyl.html; accessed April 2012

while people that have Type 1 diabetes can use the HCG diet protocol safely, the health benefits are not as dramatic as the benefits for a person with Type 2 Diabetes.

The reason why Type 2 diabetics can gain greater benefits from the HCG diet is because they are not insulin dependent. Instead, excessive weight is one of the contributing factors to this form of diabetes (T2) so losing weight is actually beneficial. Altering one's diet and getting one's weight under control is one of the disease management techniques used by many Type 2 diabetics. After speaking with a medically HCG trained physician about using the HCG dieting plan, a diabetic can begin to lose weight quickly. Rapid weight loss can lead to improved blood pressure control, less strain on the heart, and improved blood sugar levels; all of which are of great concern to the individual that suffers from Type 2 diabetes.

The HCG diet plan, when used correctly, can reduce blood glucose levels in a matter of days. As the diet progresses, glucose levels continue to decline until they eventually return to normal levels in the body: this can happen over the course of 1- 2 weeks.

If you are interested in HCG diet plans please avoid homeopathic HCG as this is a total fraud. I am a trained Homeopath and would not use homeopathic HCG to induce weight loss. When Dr Simeons was researching the HCG protocol he used *real* HCG, not homeopathic HCG. There are many businesses toting Homeopathic HCG for weight loss who give a free copy of Simeon's book to authenticate the sale. DO NOT trust homeopathic HCG. Fortunately the FDA has now started proceedings to ban homeopathic HCG for weight loss.

Only *real* HCG will work to raise the hormone levels of testosterone and progesterone. That's the key; the hormones raise the fat burn factor.

A good organization that deals with the training of physicians in the HCG protocol is IAPAM of the USA. Having trained with them, I practice the detail needed on a biochemistry level to guide patients precisely during the fat reduction process through the HCG diet. Maxing the biochemistry to create the best safe fat burn.

Diabetes goes into remission with the HCG diet due to the:

1. Very Low calories for a few weeks.
2. Hormone boost to help burn fat.
3. Boosted hormones improve insulin sensitivity.
4. Fat cells, which block the pancreas secretions, are unplugged.
5. Maintenance phase of the diet allows for a new set weight point.

Please find a local clinic to guide you through this process if you want rapid weight loss at the same time as reversing your type 2 diabetes. Instructions for this are beyond the scope of this book and are covered in my other book 'The Total Fat Cure', but the principle is that lower carbohydrates allow a good fat burn and diabetic recovery, particularly if you can boost your own hormones. The massive fat burn unplugs all the fat residues around the pancreas that inhibit the proper release of insulin.

This 'staged' fat burn through lower calories (low Glycemic Index foods) and extra natural hormones reboots the metabolism of the body.

8. Avoiding Diabetic Complications

There are two ways to avoid diabetic complications:
1) Use a medical team

Using a medical team such as your Doctor, Osteopath, Podiatrist, Nutritionist/ dietician and personal trainer are key to getting successful improvements in diabetic problems.

Your physician will help guide you through the process of recovery in terms of medication management and prescription reductions. MD's are the only ones who are legally allowed to do this.

Podiatrists will look after your very important feet and a good nutritionist will help with your food choices and supplementation.

2) Choose a Low GI Diet for Life

Together with the information in this book your dietician or nutritionist will guide the nutrition process for you based on the Glycemic Index[114]. If

---

114 Jennie Brand-Miller, PhD, Susan Hayne, BSc, Peter Petocz, PhD and Stephen Colagiuri, MD. Low–Glycemic Index Diets in the Management of Diabetes. A meta-analysis of randomized controlled trials Diabetes Care August 2003 vol. 26 no. 8 2261-2267

one can get this achieved then one can avoid all the diabetic complications because exercise and diet are proven techniques to reduce blood pressure, improve circulation and reverse Type 2 diabetes.

Remember a good nutritionist will help you remove unhealthy carbohydrates, wheat, and all sugars. If they do not do this you are in the wrong nutritionist's office.

Diabetic complications are frequently understated. The complications are due to the person not drastically reducing the carbohydrate intake. Not many people know the extent to which these complications ruin the quality of life of a diabetic, the immediate family in terms of emotional stress and society in general.

Diabetics do not die from diabetes but from their complications[115]. Diabetics endure high blood pressure, progressive blindness and heart problems; and if that's not enough they also sometimes have to witness their toes or feet being amputated. This is extremely stressful and can cause depression.

Even when diabetics are taking their medications so that the glucose stays strictly within the reference range, a large percentage will still suffer from complications such as heart disease, kidney disease, foot disorders, eye disease and cancer. What's more, in 2004 the American Diabetic Association stated that over 68% of the complications that resulted in death are heart attack related and a further 16% resulted in stroke[116].

It is the diabetic complications that end up killing the patient. Diabetes is 90% preventable[117,118] and yet so many people end up with diabetes and the associated complications due to a lack of education and discipline about controlling their diet.

So the best thing you can do right now in order to lower the risk of

---

[115] Saleh N, Petursson P, Lagerqvist B, Skúladóttir H, Svensson A, Eliasson B, Gudbjörnsdottir S, Eeg-Olofsson K, Norhammar A. Long-term mortality in patients with type 2 diabetes undergoing coronary angiography: the impact of glucose-lowering treatment. Diabetologia. 2012 May 8.
[116] Data from the 2011 National Diabetes Fact Sheet (released Jan. 26, 2011). http://www.diabetes.org/diabetes-basics/diabetes-statistics. Accessed 2012
[117] Summaries for patients. Improving each additional lifestyle factor further reduces the risk for diabetes. Ann Intern Med. 2011 Sep 6;155(5):292-9.
[118] *Mozaffarian D, Kamineni A, Carnethon M, Djoussé L, Mukamal KJ, Siscovick D.*Lifestyle risk factors and new-onset diabetes mellitus in older adults: the cardiovascular health study. *Arch Intern Med. 2009 Apr 27; 169(8):798-807.*

diabetic complications is to lower your carbohydrate intake[119], make sure you choose low Glycemic Index carbohydrates (<50) and take an anti-fungal capsule to encourage the remission of yeast[120].

The Newcastle University Study adds to the proof that diabetes & obesity are diseases with a defined pathology, which can be controlled by extreme changes in calorie intake, even for one week.

As the percentage of the global population with diabetes & obesity continues to increase[121], the Newcastle University study by Prof. Roy Taylor clarifies the health risk of the high-calorie diets we have come to accept as the norm. It may also highlight the current distorted view of how many calories an average person needs in a day, especially older adults.

---

119 Zhu S, St-Onge MP, Heshka S, Heymsfield SB.,Lifestyle behaviors associated with lower risk of having the metabolic syndrome. Metabolism. 2004 Nov;53(11):1503- 1511------. http://www.ncbi.nlm.nih.gov/pubmed/15536610
120 Costantini, AV, *Fungalbionics Series; Etiology and Prevention of Atherosclerosis*. Johann Freidrich Oberlin Verlag. Freiburg, Germany. 1998/99. Chp. 17, pg 71-76
121 Mokdad AH, Bowman BA, Ford ES, Vinicor F, Marks JS, Koplan JP. The continuing epidemics of obesity and diabetes in the united states. JAMA. 2001;286(10):1195-1200.

Step 1

Learn about Carbohydrates

What do you need to do in order to get diabetes to go into remission?
Health Tip:
Eat Less Carbs / Sugar[1] & More Protein

- Eat less carbs and sugar[2], and replace with more protein.
- ALWAYS eat a carb with a protein; ratio of 1:1->2 (carbs, Gly' index dependent).
- Women: restrict sugars to less than 20-45 grams per meal.
- Men: restrict sugars to 45-60 grams per meal.
- No soft drinks. No alcohol.
- Eat no foods with yeast; for instance, white bread or white rice.
- Eat only complex carbohydrates (Yams / cassava / ground foods).
- Lower your calorie count to aid weight loss and diabetic (T2) reversal.

Definition of Diabetes

> *"Diabetes is a medical disorder producing excessive urine and high blood sugar levels."*

Diabetes is a disease in which your blood glucose or sugar levels are too high. Glucose comes from the foods that you consume.

Diabetes is as 'old as the hills' and has been around for centuries. Ancient

---

[1] Gannon M, Nutall F. Effect of A High-Protein , low carbohydrate Diet on Blood Glucose in people with Type 2 Diabetes. DIABETES, Vol.53 2375 – 2382, sept. 2004 -
[2] Gannon M, Nutall F. Effect of A High-Protein , low carbohydrate Diet on Blood Glucose in people with Type 2 Diabetes. DIABETES, Vol.53 2375 – 2382, sept. 2004 -

physicians both in Egypt and Greece were aware of this rare disease; however, they did not recognize then that it was a disease related to a diseased pancreas.

The Greek physician Aretaeus coined the term 'Diabetes' in the first century AD, which means, 'siphon' due to the excessive urination. The early physicians of Greece could not treat diabetes and so the patients slowly wasted away through over peeing.

Diabetes is today one of the fastest growing epidemics in the world and is responsible for killing approximately 5% of the world's population. Poor diets can cause the body to over-produce insulin, which in turn creates the deposition of fat cells.

The effect of high long-term insulin levels is weight gain and obesity. As people get fatter they develop a chronic condition called Hyper-insulinemia, which means that the pancreas secretes way too much insulin and the body is unable to use it properly. This creates a constant feeling of hunger in the body, and this in turn results in the development of a vicious circle.

Increased hunger causes more simple carbohydrates to be eaten, which causes weight gain and further insulin dysregulation. Of course any latent fungal infection will enjoy and reinforce this type of food behavior. (More on this later.) Unfortunately diabetics are prone to yeast/fungal infections as fungi love sugar, and these are usually higher in a diabetic human.

How does sugar cause diabetes?

Sugar in large amounts causes inflammation and suppresses the immune system. Too much sugar in the diet will cause the dysregulation of the body's sugar feedback mechanism and cause an insensitive state called *insulin resistance*. This causes more sugar to be left in the blood stream, which in turn causes more inflammation. Chronic Inflammation causes chronic degenerative disease.

Research has shown that patients will progress through a series of phases of insulin resistance and glucose sensitivity before becoming a classic type 2 diabetic. The stages are as follows:

- **Hypoglycemia** – blood sugar dropping too low.
- **Insulin Resistance** – fatigue, brain fog, poor memory, gas and bloating,

sleepiness after a meal, depression, hair-loss, high blood pressure, heart disease, obesity, kidney diseases and cancer.
- **Diabetes** - Type 1 (Insulin dependent) and Type 2 (non-insulin dependent) – hyperglycemia.

So what happens if one eats too much sugar, too regularly?

Well the sensitivity of the fat cells that are storing the sugar as fat, get progressively numb. They become less sensitive to the calling of the insulin and they, therefore, let the sugars remain in the blood stream. This then sets up a domino effect that causes the pancreas to secrete even more insulin.

As the blood levels of sugar remain high over time, the fat cells lose their ability to respond to the insulin signal and the pancreas works harder and harder to meet the demands of the sugar regulation; the fat cell's reception becomes more insensitive and the islet cells start to die. This is the start of insulin resistance and, eventually, Type 2 diabetes.

Diabetes involves carbohydrates such as glucose, fructose, and sucrose. The majority of our food choices revolve around these sugars in the form of candy, bread, potatoes, milk shakes, chocolates, fruits and pastries. People who eat too many of these foods are setting themselves up for problems in years to come.

Relying on prescription medication to solve a bad diet is not the answer.

Choosing the right carbohydrate foods that contain a low Glycemic Index is the right answer to this problem.

Once you have received the diagnosis of Type 2 diabetes, it is very likely that you have lost 60-80 % of your insulin producing cells. Those precious islet cells have either died or become dysfunctional and these are the cells that produce your insulin. For this reason you must look after the remaining 20-40% as best as possible.

How do you do this?

By having the knowledge as to how much sugar or carbohydrate is in each food item *BEFORE* you eat it you will be able to make informed choices to guide your sugar back to its optimum level. This is known as the Glycemic Index (GI).

Before you eat a meal you must ensure that the GI of your food choice is correct and falls under 50 on the GI scale.

There is a list of the GI indexes of foods in the appendix of this book.

With each low GI meal the blood sugar will stabilize lower and lower, slowly moving lower, two-ten points at a time. You will know that the program is working because after a couple of meals / days your fasting blood sugar levels will get closer to the optimal ranges of 80-100 mg/dl.

Action Steps:

Control the carbohydrates in your meal by:

1. Choose low Glycemic Index foods.
2. Avoid all sugar and high fructose corn syrup (HFCS).
3. Heal your pancreas with specific natural substances such as foods, good fats and vitamins.
4. Stop the diabetic domino effect.
5. Get organized and build your medical recovery team, with your MD and Osteopath, dietician, and personal trainer.[3]

The Glycemic Index (GI) - Slow Carbohydrates and Fast Carbohydrates

For a full list of the GI indexes of foods please see the appendix.

Not all carbohydrates are created equal. Some carbohydrates have a little glucose in them and some have a lot. The Higher GI carbohydrates (fast carbohydrates) are linked to chronic degenerative diseases. The Lower GI carbohydrates (the slow carbohydrates) are linked to improved blood sugar function[4], less inflammation and longevity.

---

3 http://articles.mercola.com/sites/articles/archive/2001/05/12/diabetes-part-two.aspx
4 Manny Noakes, Paul R Foster, Jennifer B Keogh, Anthony P James, John C Mamo and Peter M Clifton. Comparison of isocaloric very low carbohydrate/high saturated fat and high carbohydrate/low saturated fat diets on body composition and cardiovascular risk. *Nutrition & Metabolism* 2006, 3:7 Published: 11 January 2006

Obesity and Type 2 diabetes are at epidemic levels[5] in the 21st century and science is now telling us that in order to avoid serious degenerative diseases we should choose wisely as to what carbohydrate choices we make at meal times and snacks.

According to the WHO's Prof. Costantini, the retired head of the WHO Collaboration Centre for Mycotoxins in Foods, fungi exploit humans by feeding off the sugars that humans consume. Today in our modern society many popular foods and snacks are laced with ever increasing amounts of sugar or high fructose corn syrup (fast carbohydrates). These will cause weight gain in an individual that does not exercise regularly.

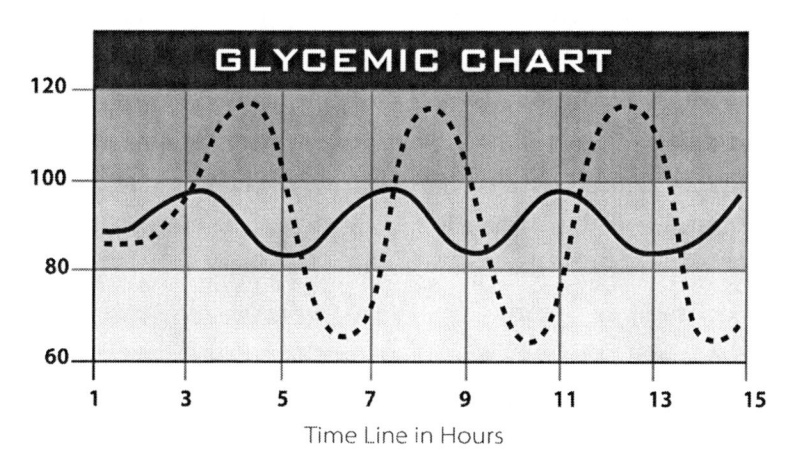

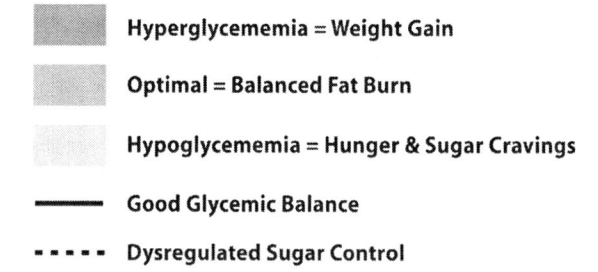

GLYCEMIC CHART

Time Line in Hours

- **Hyperglycememia = Weight Gain**
- **Optimal = Balanced Fat Burn**
- **Hypoglycememia = Hunger & Sugar Cravings**
- **Good Glycemic Balance**
- **Dysregulated Sugar Control**

---

5   Lee S Gross, Li Li, Earl S Ford and Simin Liu Increased consumption of refined carbohydrates and the epidemic of type 2 diabetes in the United States: an ecologic assessment. Am J Clin Nutr May 2004 vol. 79 no. 5 774-779

If you look at the above chart, the dashed line is the result of somebody eating a high GI food. The blood sugar will rise sharply, causing weight gain and then it is soon followed by a crash that induces *hunger and sugar cravings*.

This is a trap and a vicious circle. Up to the sugar mountain (fat) and then a free gift pass down into the sugar valley (hunger). Get fat and then get hungry. Get fat and then get hungry ! That's a crazy disease inducing loop that a lot of Americans and Brits and the rest of the world is caught in.

The food companies know it too. Sugar is addictive and it sells. It's like legal crack. Whitney Houston said "crack is whack" so what's sugar?

Sugar is thwack. A really sharp blow to the body every time it's is eaten in excess levels. Punching that pancreas, bruising it for years until it can deal with the onslaught no more. It tries to protect itself by turning sugar into fat and deal with it another day.

Fast carbohydrates will cause your body to store the unused energy in the food as fat. If that individual has a current yeast infection, a slow thyroid, or sluggish adrenal glands, the effect is a huge escalation in weight. It is this theory that accounts for the obesity levels we see today.

Xylose sugar or erythritol are natural sugar alcohols[6], used as a sugar substitute is well tolerated[7], which has been approved for use in the USA and throughout much of the world. Xylose sugar occurs naturally in fruits, birch trees and corncobs. It has a low GI and is used successfully with Candida sufferers[8], diabetics, cholesterol patients and patients who are concerned with weight-loss or who are simply health conscious.

Xylose has a mild laxative effect (which is an advantage sometimes to relieve constipation) whereas erythritol does not cause any loosening of the bowels. The GI of Xylitol is seven. The GI of sugar is 100.

As I have stated in my first book '*The Hidden Cure*', the GI value is im-

---

6   Martí, N.; Funes, L.L.; Saura, D.; Micol, V. (July 2008). "An update on alternative sweeteners". *International sugar journal* 110 (1315): 425–429.
7   Mäkinen, KK (1976). "Long-term tolerance of healthy human subjects to high amounts of xylitol and fructose: general and biochemical findings". *Internationale Zeitschrift fur Vitamin und Ernahrungsforschung Beiheft* 15: 92–104
8   Abu-Elteen, Khaled H. (2005). "The influence of dietary carbohydrates on adherence of four species to human buccal epithelial cells". *Microbial Ecology in Health and Disease* 17 (3): 156–162.

portant because if foods are chosen that are high on the GI scale, they will cause *the body to store excess sugar as fat.*

In this day and age of abundant carbohydrates, the human ability to store carbohydrates as fat is now effectively killing people through modern degenerative diseases such as diabetes, heart disease, cancer, hypertension and depression. Sadly, hundreds of thousands of lives will be wasted every year because of excessive fat build up and the consequential diseases that ensue.

The wisest thing to do while we are all set in this backdrop of having chronic degenerative diseases is to actively resist the fungi's craving for fast carbohydrates and move towards a healthier option of slow carbohydrate choices.

What will the results be like?

What will happen if you apply this information is nothing short of liberating.

Patients typically lose weight, lower their blood pressure and have way more energy than they did before. All the symptoms of diabetes Type 2 will reverse. You will live longer than if you hadn't done anything about it.

You will probably need to wear smaller clothing, take fewer medications and generally become way more social and fun to hang out with as your self-esteem and energy will also improve - especially if the program has been extended for one - two months.

Step 2

Learn about Proteins

Eat right for your blood type.

In my clinic, proteins must be chosen according to *Paleo-blood type* theory and should, preferably, be organic and free from hormones and antibiotics.

Paleo-blood type theory: scientists have put forward a report recently in the British Journal of Nutrition that gives a scientific modernized approximation of what diet our "caveman" ancestors may have eaten throughout time, starting as far back as their initial emergence in Africa some 200,000 years ago[1].

The Paleo-blood type approach has been compared to the Mediterranean Diet and has shown that it is better at improving metabolism[2] and cardiovascular function overall[3]. The report shows that our ancestors ate higher percentages of protein, in the region of 25-29%, 40 % carbs and 30 % fats. Our Paleo ancestors consumed the Omega oils, according to the report, in relatively moderate amounts approx. 6-grams/ day in the form of wild game & fish. This is a very similar ratio to the protein metabolic type which you will read about in the next chapter.

---

1 Kuipers RS, Luxwolda MF, Dijck-Brouwer DJA, Eaton SB, Crawford, MA, Cordain L, and Muskiet FAJ. *"Estimate macronutrient and fatty acid intakes from an East African paleolithic diet."* British J Nutr 104: 1666-1687 (2010)
2 Frassetto LA, Schloetter M, Mietus-Synder M, Morris RC, and Sebastian A. *"Metabolic and physiologic improvements from consuming a Paleolithic, hunter-gatherer type diet."* Eur J Clin Nutr 63: 947-955 (2009)
3 Lindberg S, Jonsson T, Granfeldt Y, Borgstrand E, Soffman J, Sjorstrom K, and Ahren B. *"A Paleolithic diet improves glucose tolerance more than a Mediterranean-like diet in individuals with ischaemic heart disease."* Diabetologia 50: 1795-1807 (2007)

When one starts to eat this way, one will experience an immediate shift in metabolism and consequential weight loss especially in a T2 Diabetic[4]. This will also happen in patients who are healthy and have no T2 Diabetes[5].

Please see the appendix for a list of Paleo-blood type appropriate protein choices.

- Beef
- Chicken
- Turkey
- Ostrich
- Cornish hens
- Eggs
- Rabbit
- Fish
- Lamb & mutton

What are the effects of eating the wrong Proteins?

In my professional opinion, eating the wrong proteins according to Paleo-blood type will cause inflammation, digestive disorders and allergies (IgA, IgE IgG etc). This will burden your immune system, leading to abnormal levels of Cortisol, which leads to the premature burnout of the adrenals. Weak adrenals can induce a functional disturbance within the pancreas because Cortisol disturbs blood sugar regulation.

In my practice, I have advised patients to follow blood type theory because my experience and observations over 15 years have indicated that certain blood types do not do well with certain proteins e.g. O bloods, for instance, have an issue with wheat and dairy, A's have an issue with red meat and are usually the best vegetarians, B bloods are usually allergic to shrimp / shellfish / chicken and lastly AB's have issues with red meat / chicken and shellfish, but can also be good vegetarians. The jury is still out on this, but

---
[4] Markovic TP, Jenkins AB, Campbell LV, Furler SM, Kragen EW, and Chisholm DJ. *"The determinants of Glycemic responses to diet restriction and weight loss in obesity and NI-DDM."* Diabetes Care 21: 687-694 (1998)
[5] Osterdahl M. Kocturk T. Koochek A, and Wandell PE. *"Effects of a short-term intervention with a Paleolithic diet in healthy volunteers."* Eur J Clin Nutr 62: 682-685 (2008)

I share my observations of patients with you so that you might also see the same trends.

What is Blood Type Theory?

The theory of blood type and diet has been thoroughly explored and go along the lines of correct diet based on ancestral lineage. Numerous research articles about ethno-paleontology have led to the Paleolithic diet[6] and the 'eat right for your blood type'[7] diet. It is a loose theory and is used merely as a guide for the proteins my patients at my clinic are advised to eat. Eating protein rich foods over carbs stabilizes insulin in humans[8]. Records show that agriculture was a recent invention by humans dating around the end of the last age. The mass production of cereals (carbs), due to a growing demand of an increasing urban population, led to a decline in overall health[9]. There is some evidence that our bodies are still adjusting (in the form of chronic disease) from the shift in dietary trends from meat eaters to plants eaters. In a research study written in the American Journal of Clinical Nutrition[10], the authors point to the fact that:

> *In the United States and most Western countries, diet-related chronic diseases represent the single largest cause of morbidity and mortality. These diseases are epidemic in contemporary Westernized populations and typically afflict 50–65% of the adult population, yet they are rare or nonexistent in hunter-gatherers and other less Westernized people.*

In our clinic, the 2nd step to curing your diabetes is about the blood type and how to get the right type and amount of protein as determined by

---

6 Voegtlin, Walter L. (1975). *The stone age diet: Based on in-depth studies of human ecology and the diet of man*. Vantage Press. ISBN 0-533-01314-3.
7 D'Adamo, P. (with additional material by Catherine Whitney) (1996). *Eat Right 4 your Type*. Putnam. ISBN 0-399-14255-X
8 Lindeberg S, Eliasson M, Lindahl B, Ahrén B (October 1999). "Low serum insulin in traditional Pacific Islanders—The Kitava study". *Metabolism* 48 (10): 1216–19.
9 Eaton, S. Boyd; Cordain, Loren; & Sebastian, Anthony (2007). *"The Ancestral Biomedical Environment* (PDF)". In Aird, William C.. *Endothelial Biomedicine*. Cambridge University Press. pp. 129–34
10 Loren Cordain, S Boyd Eaton, Anthony Sebastian, Neil Mann, Staffan Lindeberg, Bruce A Watkins, James H O'Keefe and Janette Brand-Miller, *Origins and evolution of the Western diet: health implications for the 21st century*. Am J Clin Nutr February 2005 vol. 81 no. 2 341-354

an individual's blood type and body weight, respectively. The theory is that if one eats the wrong protein, it can create a "shift" in the pH of the blood and this in turn creates allergies and lowered oxygen levels within the blood, setting up a Rouleaux effect[11]. Rouleaux involves the stacking and sticking of the red blood cells.

As one can imagine, this effect creates a sluggish flow and a lack of oxygen within the body. One can see this clearly under the microscope, where it tells a fascinating story about one's diet and lifestyle choices. While healthy individuals have great flowing blood, sick people have poor flowing blood. Improvements can be seen when the patient follows the blood type protein law.

Step 2 action steps:

Please refer to the appendix for specific guidelines on blood type and protein choices from the shopping list.

Summary of Blood Types

Below is a brief interpretation of Dr. D'Adamo's work on blood types. For more insight into this exciting field of naturopathy, please refer to his work Eat Right for your Blood Type[12] blended with the Paleo-diet.

Type O Blood, 44 Percent of the Global Population

The Stone Age caveman diet suits O bloods the best, in my opinion. The blood group O is the original hunter-gatherer bloodstock. This blood type developed in a strong and tough environment and theoretically originates from Africa. Animal flesh, bird meats and fish were the predominant protein source at the time, and through evolution, these blood types adapted to the amount and type of protein, producing a lot of stomach acid to break it down. O bloods historically have a high incidence of stomach ulcers and gastritis from the over-secretion of gastric acid.

---

11   Iwona Cicha, Yoji Suzuki, Norihiko Tateishi, and Nobuji Maeda, *Changes of RBC aggregation in oxygenation-deoxygenation: pH dependency and cell morphology,* AJP - Heart June 1, 2003 vol. 284 no. 6 H2335-H2342

12   D'Adamo, P. (with additional material by Catherine Whitney) (1996). *Eat Right 4 your Type.* Putnam. ISBN 0-399-14255-X

O bloods should avoid farm-based protein foods, such as wheat and dairy as these are allergic food proteins. O bloods have strong immune systems and constitutions with a very efficient metabolism. Their risks are clotting disorders, and they tend to have slow thyroids, hence kelp or seaweed for its strong iodine content is beneficial. O's benefit from intense physical exercise to stay healthy.

General supplements for O's:

- B vitamins
- Iodine (thyroid)
- Licorice (caution with high blood pressure; use instead deglycyrrhized licorice DGL)
- Calcium carbonate (to offset general acidity)
- Kelp/seaweed
- Vitamin K

Type-A Blood, 40 Percent of Global Population

The next in line on the evolutionary tree are the A bloods (agrarians), and the general location for their development was the Middle East, India and Southern Asia (all areas south of the Silk Road). These have adapted to eating grains and beans especially soy and soy products, making soy very beneficial for this blood group. The DNA shift from O meat eating to A plant/harvesting coincided with the agricultural revolution, and the controlled systematic planting of seeds for harvesting. A bloods are the agriculturists.

A bloods are the most vegetarian of the blood types, but they still benefit from occasional fish, turkey, and chicken. This blood group produces less stomach acid, because traditionally they did not eat complex proteins such as red meat. Exercise should consist of calming, stretching exercises such as walking, yoga, and Pilates.

General supplements for A's:

- Vitamin B12
- Folic acid

- Vitamin C
- Vitamin E
- Milk thistle
- Echinacea

Type-B Blood, 11 Percent of Global Population

This blood group developed in North Asia, from Mongolia to China, north of the Silk Road. D'Adamo regards these as the nomads. The B blood's have a strong immune system and are very versatile and adaptable. B's developed in difficult, colder climates and have a wide variety of food choices. This group can tolerate dairy in large amounts and they have no natural weaknesses except a tendency towards autoimmune diseases. This blood group, being landlocked in evolutionary terms, is allergic to shrimp and other shellfish. They should also avoid chicken and other poultry, as this produces a dangerous lectin response. They enjoy moderate exercise such as cross training, aerobics, and swimming.

General supplements for B's:

- Magnesium
- Licorice or DGL
- Gingko biloba
- Lecithin

AB Blood, 5 Percent of Global Population

This is the youngest of the blood groups. This blood group evolved from the mixing of B types and A types along the Great Silk Road, the major trade route between the East and West in early human history. AB's are suited to contemporary lifestyles and have very strong immune systems. They carry the benefits of both A's and B's but should still avoid shellfish and chicken.

General supplements for AB's:

- Vitamin C
- Echinacea

- Milk thistle
- Valerian root
- Hawthorne berry

Why the Correct Amount of Protein

Key Points:

- Carbohydrates cause an increase insulin output. Insulin promotes the storage of sugar/carbs into FAT
- Protein causes increased glucagon output. Glucagon promotes mobilization and utilization of stored fat to convert into glucose / energy.

When one eats excess carbohydrates we produce excessive levels of insulin and little glucagon. When we eat more protein we secrete more glucagon, which in turn causes us to become more thermogenic (fat-burn) and lose weight[13].

The amount of protein to ingest is often overlooked in people's diets, and under-calculating it can result in a tendency to foster weight gain and build fat, which can in turn cause fermentation. However, a high protein diet has greater health advantages over a high carb diet when treating diabetic and obese patients[14,15]. One must keep the following two guidelines in mind:

Protein needs to be adequately chewed and digested. Too much protein can overload the digestive system, which only causes more rotting within the system (check albumen levels to indicate stomach acid sufficiency on a blood test). Most books on nutrition suggest three to five ounces of protein per day for an average adult.

If one wants to lose weight, my suggestion is always to increase protein and decrease carbohydrates intake (please refer to Table 6.1 below for approx-

---

13   Baba NH, Sawaya S, Torbay N, Habbal Z, Azar S, Hashim SA, *High protein vs high carbohydrate hypoenergetic diet for the treatment of obese hyperinsulinemic subjects., International journal of obesity and related metabolic disorders* : Journal of the International Association for the Study of Obesity [1999, 23(11):1202-6]
14   Ibid 13.
15   Barkeling B, Rossner S, Bjorvell H: *Effects of a high-protein meal (meat) and a high-carbohydrate meal (vegetarian) on satiety measured by automated computerized monitoring of subsequent food intake, motivation to eat and food preferences.* Int J Obes 14: 743–751, 1990

imate amounts). As one increases protein and decreases carbohydrates intake, one could supplement with more vegetables and salads to fill the stomach. This is an important adjustment to the dietary strategy.

The chart that follows is the recommended **amount of protein per day** intake that I suggest to my patients at my clinic.

- One or more of the meals should definitely consist of proteins. The rest can comprise of mixed salads, vegetables, and low GI starch ground provisions such as eddoes, pumpkin, squash, cassava (yucca), or yam.
- Dinner should always be lighter than lunch as the body is winding down its metabolism. Therefore, it is recommended to eat salads, steamed or stir-fry vegetables, and a little serving of ground provisions with the right amount of protein for the height of the body.
- Athletes and pregnant women need to eat much larger amounts of protein as both are highly anabolic and have much faster metabolisms compared to ordinary adult metabolisms.
- Be sensible and choose the right amount of protein. High protein diets should be avoided in patients with kidney issues[16][17].
- If you want to build muscle, burn fat[18] [19] and reduce carb cravings[20][21] use more proteins, less carbohydrates and lots of vegetables and salads.
- Satiety was markedly increased with the high-protein diet. The reverse

---

16 Skov AR, Toubro S, Bulow J, Krabbe K, Parving HH, Astrup A: *Changes in renal function during weight loss induced by high vs. low-protein low-fat diets in overweight subjects.* Int J Obes 23: 1170–1177, 1999

17 Brändle E, Sieberth HG, Hautmann RE: *Effect of chronic dietary protein intake on the renal function in healthy subjects.* Eur J Clin Nutr 50: 734–740, 1996.

18 Emma Farnsworth, Natalie D Luscombe, Manny Noakes, Gary Wittert, Eleni Argyiou and Peter M Clifton. *Effect of a high-protein, energy-restricted diet on body composition, Glycemic control, and lipid concentrations in overweight and obese hyperinsulinemic men and women.* Am J Clin Nutr July 2003 vol. 78 no. 1 31-39

19 Carol S. Johnston, PhD, FACN, Carol S. Day, MS and Pamela D. Swan, PhD *Postprandial Thermogenesis Is Increased 100% on a High-Protein, Low-Fat Diet versus a High-Carbohydrate, Low-Fat Diet in Healthy, Young Women,* J Am Coll Nutr February 2002 vol. 21 no. 1 55-61

20 Baba NH, Sawaya S, Torbay N, Habbal Z, Azar S, Hashim SA, *High protein vs high carbohydrate hypoenergetic diet for the treatment of obese hyperinsulinemic subjects., International journal of obesity and related metabolic disorders* : journal of the International Association for the Study of Obesity [1999, 23(11):1202-6]

21 Arne Astrup .The satiating power of protein—a key to obesity prevention? Am J Clin Nutr 2005 82: 1-2

is also true in that if you want to build fat, eat more carbohydrates and less protein, and experience cravings.

Table of Protein/ day Quantities as Related to Height[22]
Note: 1 oz = 28 g

Height	5'2–5'6	5'6–5'10	5'10–6'2
Male Adult	4-5-6 oz	6-7-8 oz	7–8–9 oz
Female Adult	4-5-6 oz	6-7oz	6.5-7-8 oz

What if?

If you apply this information about the correct protein choices you will feel so much better as you will have less allergies and the start of a stronger immune system.

If you don't apply this information then you can expect continued allergy and inflammatory diseases in your life.

---

22 Clinical Observations. The Maas Clinic, Barbados 1997 - 2012

Step 3

Burning Fats According to Your Metabolic Type

We have already covered the 1st law in chapter one; get the right carbohydrates into your body. The 2nd law is to select the correct proteins (type and amount). Now it's time to learn about the good fats in our diet and how we can shift our "fat" metabolism by eating according to our metabolic type.

Good "fats" usually come in three forms:

1. Dairy
2. Fats – animal / vegetable
3. Oils – fish / seeds / nuts

Dairy - Consider using organic sources and follow the blood-type rules for dairy, as it is considered a partial protein (dairy also contains fats). If you are allergic to wheat or gluten, dairy will have to be omitted for at least two weeks. After two weeks, have a piece of cheese or glass of milk and see if there is a gas or bloating reaction. If there was a reaction then avoid consuming dairy.

Apply blood type rules well; for example, only B and AB are allowed cow's milk and O bloods must use dairy sparingly. If unsure, check for allergies by doing an allergy test both IgE and IgG.

- Butter, ghee
- Goat's cheese

- Feta cheese
- Mozzarella
- Ricotta
- Yoghurt (live acidophilus)
- Cottage cheese
- Milk (organic cows or goats)
- Milk beverages (soy or almond are replacements for dairy milk)

Fats and Oils – Our Paleo blood type ancestors would eat approximately 30% fats and oils in their diet[1].

- Fish oils
- Flax seed oil
- Hemp oil
- Coconut oil
- Olive oil
- Mayonnaise
- Avocado
- Meat / animal fat
- Egg yolks

Why metabolism?

To "burn fat" you need to understand what your metabolism is doing and choose the appropriate food ratios of Protein & Fats Vs Carbs to match.

If you don't do this, then certain fatty foods that you eat could slow you down or speed you up. No guesswork, find out what your metabolic type is and then you can choose the right food ratios to help nudge your metabolism for the better.

NB. Hydrogenated fats and trans-fatty acids as well as Canola oil are to be avoided as they can harm the body.

---

1 Kuipers RS, Luxwolda MF, Dijck-Brouwer DJA, Eaton SB, Crawford, MA, Cordain L, and Muskiet FAJ. *"Estimate macronutrient and fatty acid intakes from an East African paleolithic diet."* British J Nutr 104: 1666-1687 (2010)

What is Metabolic Typing?

Metabolic Typing is a method of evaluating, and interpreting your metabolism to determine what your individual reaction is to foods and nutrients. We all inherit strengths and weaknesses i.e. definite gene patterns of biological and neurological origin that decide our personal nutritional necessities. This is based on the work of William Walcott[2]. If one corrects the metabolic imbalance by choosing the right ratios of food then fat will be burnt.

Eating by Metabolic Typing

In this chapter, I will introduce you to the concept of metabolic type. I had mentioned this in my previous book 'The Hidden Cure'; however, I correlated it to the basic functions of the adrenal glands and thyroid gland. The adrenal glands and the thyroid gland both influence the rate at which the body metabolizes fat.

Firstly, in this chapter, I will discuss the human nervous system a little deeper and how it plays a role in our metabolism (i.e. how fast we burn off fat). In 1919 Francis M. Pottenger, M.D. originally put this clinical model forward. He explained that he thought all organs and glands in the body are connected to the brain (hypothalamus) via the Autonomic Nervous System (ANS).

ANS controls the involuntary activities of the body (i.e. heart rate, blood pressure, digestion, restoring homeostasis, immune systems, metabolism etc.) ANS has two divisions: **Sympathetic and Parasympathetic** systems.

I will also show you how, through our diets, we can influence our nervous system and metabolic rate. Subsequently, I will discuss the thyroid and then the adrenals and how we can use certain supplements to help rebuild our thyroid and adrenal glands in order to increase our metabolic energy.

---

[2] Wiiliam Walcott & Trish Fahey, *The Metabolic Typing Diet: Customize Your Diet to Your Own Unique Body Chemistry*- Three Rivers Press; 1st Bway Bks Tr Ppbk Ed 2002 edition (January 2, 2002)

Metabolic Type Quiz Analysis

The ideas and Techniques in this section are, primarily, to do with fat metabolism (or fat burn); however, it will also be important for you to work out whether you are a protein or a carbohydrate type (i.e. whether your body needs to eat more carbohydrate foods or protein foods). If you are a protein type, you will enjoy eating healthy fats with your proteins and if you are a carbohydrate type, you will enjoy eating healthy fats with your carbohydrates.

No single diet works well with everyone and the same foods that keep your best friend or spouse trim, slim or thin can wind up causing you to become fat or overweight, and possibly diabetic. The key element in this equation is the autonomic nervous system (ANS), which can be either sympathetic, parasympathetic or balanced; in other words, over-stimulated or under-stimulated?

How do you work out if you are a protein (Parasympathetic) or a carbohydrate (Sympathetic) type?

BLOOD PRESSURE.

To work out if you are a sympathetic (carbohydrate) or parasympathetic (protein) type, you must look at your blood pressure.

(NB this is not appropriate for patients currently taking medication for their hypertension. These patients must see their physician before starting this.).

For this home assessment, you need to have a good **blood pressure monitor**. However, using a physician-based monitor is far better than the home digital electronic monitors. This is because home monitors only give broad readings, whilst physician-based monitors give an accurate acoustic assessment of blood pressure. Physicians use a stethoscope and sphygmanometer.

The blood pressure must be taken sitting in a relaxed mode and position.

The differential can then be worked out. The differential will be the difference between the systolic blood pressure number and the diastolic.

For instance, an average blood pressure is 120/80, which makes the differential 40. (120-80=40) The scale of the blood pressure difference will dictate the tendency.

Burning Fats According to Your Metabolic Type

1. Take your blood pressure whilst resting = __ /__
2. Subtract your systolic blood pressure from your diastolic =___
3. If the difference is greater than > 46 you are sympathetic (a carbohydrate type). If the difference is less than < 37 you are parasympathetic (a protein type)
4. If the difference is somewhere in the middle then you are a mixed balanced type.

These two types are listed below with their tendencies:

1. **Sympathetic** - large pupil, increased temperature, increased pulse, reduced appetite, unable to relax, feverish or cold sweats, gags easily, usually a tendency to have higher blood pressure- Usually a CARBOHYDRATE TYPE.
2. **Balanced** - a healthy balance between the two states – usually relates to the MIXED TYPE.
3. **Parasympathetic** - small pupil, decreased temperature, decreased pulse, increased appetite, feels lightheaded, warm hands, muscle cramps, gag reflex slow – usually a PROTEIN / FAT TYPE.

Determining your metabolic type is very important, as it will allow you to emphasize a certain way of eating to encourage greater energy and therefore weight loss. You can also take the quiz below to reveal what your metabolic type tendency is.

Quiz: (adapted from the BioMedX training course for Physicians) Answer the following questions and circle your answer

> Y or N: Is your appetite at breakfast strong?
> Y or N: Is your appetite at lunch strong?
> Y or N: Is your appetite at dinner strong?
> Y or N: Does eating before bedtime improve your sleep?
> Y or N: Do you live to eat and not to subsist?
> Y or N: Do you get hungry in b/w meals?

Y or N: Does fasting make you feel bad?
Y or N: Do you crave salt?
Y or N: Do Fatty meals agree with you?
Y or N: Does skipping meals make you uncomfortable?
Y or N: Does meat or fish at breakfast give you more energy?
Y or N: Does meat or fish at lunch give you more energy?
Y or N: Does meat or fish at dinner give you more energy?
Y or N: Does eating meat or fatty foods restore your energy?
Y or N: Do you feel bloated after meals

Count up the total of your YES answers =
Count up the total of your NO answers =

If you have more yes's = protein and fat type
If you have more No's = carbohydrate type

NB: If you find that you have an equal amount of Y and N's then you are a mixed metabolic type.

Diagnostic Assessment of Metabolic Type and meal suggestions:

Analyze your answers and see which category your metabolic type fits into. Follow the suggestions carefully, while taking into consideration your Blood type protein rules, and the ability to choose low GI to moderate GI carbohydrates. Being able to 'juggle' these key areas of carbohydrates, proteins and fats will allow you to create any metabolism you want or any body type you want.

PROTEIN and FAT TYPE (PARASYMPATHEIC)

- 70% of the meal must be Protein and Fat, 30% low GI carbohydrates.
- You must eat protein & fat with every meal and take snacks. This helps to control blood sugar swings.
- Eat protein sources such as red meats/ dark meats, nuts/ seeds/ eggs, beans.

- You should eat often throughout the day in smaller meals (x5).
- Enjoy eating fats and oils such as butter, coconut oil, and olive oil.
- Eat moderate amounts of vegetables, artichoke, asparagus, avocado, carrots, olives, peas, squash, celery, green beans and baked beans.
- Avoid high Glycemic Index fruits and fruit juices.
- The only fruits allowed are bananas, pears (firm), berries and apricots.
- You must avoid wheat, rice and sugar based products.
- Limit your grains consumption.
- Avoid vinegar consumption. Preferably remove them all together; you could use lemon instead.

CARB TYPE (SYMPATHETIC)

- Eat 40% Proteins / Fats and 60% low GI carbohydrates each meal.
- Eat low fat proteins such as poultry or fish, (no red meat).
- Avoid dairy and butter as it is high in fat; use fats v. sparingly.
- Keep high fat foods to a minimum.
- Eat plenty of vegetables and salads.
- Rely on caffeine.
- Enjoy fruits; apples, berries, grapes, pineapples, peaches, and cherries.
- High tolerance for sweets and sugar foods.
- All grains are okay except oats.
- Eat very few Nuts and Seeds.

MIXED TYPE (balance between protein/fat/carbohydrate)

- These are individuals who require a balance of protein, carbohydrates and fats.
- Variety is key and the 'mixed type' has the broadest menu options of the metabolic types.
- Some meals will follow Protein type rules and others will follow the carbohydrate type rules.
- Mixed types are in constant flux and will sometimes have a huge appetite and then at other times will be able starve for a while.

- Mixed types must be wary of high sugary foods, as this will tip them into an acidic pattern that can cause lethargy and yeast development.

Whenever eating a meal, a mixed type has to consider which rule to follow for that meal. So in other words, do they want a lot of proteins and fat with minimal carbohydrates or do they want more carbohydrates and less proteins and fats? The person's stomach and taste buds will have the answer nearer the mealtime. Be careful with caffeine, breads and alcohol.

If you are a mixed blood type, you:

- Should eat 50% Protein and fat, and 50% carbohydrates.
- Should eat protein at every meal.
- Must eat only blood type applicable dairy.
- Choose low GI to moderate GI carbohydrates.
- Must be careful with grains.
- Must avoid bread; eat Ezekiel bread as a better option.
- Should eat fats and oils in moderate amounts.
- Should avoid alcohol, sugar and caffeine.

More Clues to Fat Burning, Ketones, and Dr. Atkins

The Atkins Diet[3] is based upon having a high fat and high protein content to each meal. Carbohydrates are virtually eliminated, and the individual will start to break down fat stores to liberate caloric energy and in doing so the body produces ketones in the urine. A ketogenic diet has been found to be beneficial in patients with epilepsy[4] in that the ketone bodies modify the functioning of the brain and nervous system[5].

Ketones are present only when the body is burning fats, or when a person is diabetic and also burning fats. In short, ketones equal fat burning. This

---

3 Atkins, Robert MD, *Dr. Atkins' New Diet Revolution*, Revised Edition M.Evans & Company; 3 Sub edition (July 29, 2002)
4 Eric H. Kossoff, MD, Gregory L. Krauss, MD, Jane R. McGrogan, RD and John M. Freeman, MD. *Efficacy of the Atkins diet as therapy for intractable epilepsy*-- Neurology December 23, 2003 vol. 61 no. 12 1789-1791
5 Sirven, J., Whedon, B., Caplan, D., Liporace, J., Glosser, D., O'Dwyer, J. and Sperling, M. R. (1999), *The Ketogenic Diet for Intractable Epilepsy in Adults: Preliminary Results*. Epilepsia, 40: 1721–1726.

is what Dr. Atkins was looking for in patients on his diet program. What he observed was that when patients reduced their carbohydrate intake, the result was better fat burning. As a result people lose weight and lower their high cholesterol. When one is burning fat, ketone bodies appear in the urine sample.

Significantly, many of his cardiovascular patients improved greatly from their heart disease and hypertension, as well as cholesterol imbalances[6]. However, most patients saw their symptoms return when they dropped off the diet and re-introduced carbohydrates.

Dr. Paula Franklin of the British United Provident Association BUPA, a U.K. based medical organization, stated that the Atkins diet had a high dropout rate[7]:

"My general feeling about the Atkins Diet is that, like anything that severely restricts your calories, you'll lose weight. In the short term, if you want to do it for two weeks and lose weight, it probably won't do you any harm," said Dr. Paula Franklin, from BUPA.

However, she warned,

"What you need to do in order to be healthy in the long term is to ensure your body has all the nutrients it needs."

So, a long-term diet that doesn't include many fruits and vegetables (i.e. the Atkins) wouldn't be good.

"If you want to be a healthy weight in the long term, the best approach is really lifestyle change," said Dr. Paula Franklin. Fad diets lure people with a quick fix cure, but, says Dr Franklin, *"there's no magic with weight loss, and unless you change both what you eat and what you do, you'll put weight back on again."*

---

6 Robert C Atkins. *Atkins for Life: The Complete Controlled Carb Program for Permanent weight Loss and Good Health* . St Martins Press, London 2003
7 http:www.bupa.co.uk/health_information/html/health_news/3000503diet.html

I believe Dr. Atkins failed to consider the *yeast* factor when devising his theories and diet strategy. Limiting the carbohydrates helped weight loss and created a reduction in cholesterol and blood pressure, as well as in cardiac symptoms; however, the yeast and fungus were still in the patient, waiting for something sweet and sugary. Once they received this sugar, they could then mount another phase of fungal growth, reinstalling the symptoms.

Drawbacks to the Atkins program were halitosis (or bad breath) and constipation, both of which do not appear if the saliva pH stays in the right zone of 6.4–6.9 and the patient has enough magnesium in the body by the way.

Evidence shows that long-term adherence to the Atkins Diet may cause kidney dysfunction from higher uric acid loading of the body tissues, gout[8], leukemia[9], diabetes[10,11] and higher blood pressure[12], which could lead to strokes and heart attacks.

Remember that if the cholesterol goes too low it could cause an increased risk of cancer[13], heart attacks[14] and hyperacidity, loss of sex drive, and abnormal neurological problems[15].

The Atkins program was suited to solid meat eaters, such as type O blood patients. The heavy red meat, pork, and chicken load would not agree

---

8   Richard J. Johnson, M.D., and Bruce A. Rideout, D.V.M., Ph.D. *Uric Acid and Diet — Insights into the Epidemic of Cardiovascular Disease*. Richard J. Johnson, M.D., and Bruce A. Rideout, D.V.M., Ph.D./ N Engl J Med 2004; 350:1071-1073March 11, 2004

9   LYNCH EC. Uric acid metabolism in proliferative diseases of the marrow. Arch Intern Med. 1962;109(6):639-653.

10   Abbas Dehghan, MD, DSC, Mandy van Hoek, MD, Eric J.G. Sijbrands, MD, PHD, Albert Hofman, MD, PhD and Jacqueline C.M. Witteman, PhD. *High Serum Uric Acid as a Novel Risk Factor for Type 2 Diabetes*
Diabetes Care. 2008;31:361-362

11   Satoru Kodama, MD, PHD et al. *Association Between Serum Uric Acid and Development of Type 2 Diabetes*Diabetes Care September 2009 vol. 32 no. 9 1737-1742

12   Richard J. Johnson, Dan I. Feig, Jaime Herrera-Acosta, Duk-Hee Kang. *Resurrection of Uric Acid as a Causal Risk Factor in Essential Hypertension. Hypertension.* 2005; 45: 18-20 Published online before print November 22, 2004

13   Zureik M, Courbon D, Ducimetiere P. Decline in serum total cholesterol and the risk of death from cancer. Epidemiology. 1997 Mar;8(2):137-43.

14   Uffe Ravnskov MD. *Fat and Cholesterol are Good for You*. GB Publishing (January 26, 2009)

15   Edwards, I. Ralph; Star, Kristina; Kiuru, Anne, *"Statins, Neuromuscular Degenerative Disease and an Amyotrophic Lateral Sclerosis-Like Syndrome," Drug Safety*, Volume 30, Number 6, 2007 , pp. 515-525(11)

with the A, and AB blood types[16], in whom high uric acid load could cause arthritis[17], hypertension and cardiovascular disease[18], diabetes and chronic yeast infections.

What are ketones?

Ketones are produced when you burn fats and this will usually happen when the glucose comes under control. It is key to find out if your urine contains Ketones. The more ketones, the greater the fat burn. When patients do the HCG diet with real HCG they create a really good fat burn losing up to 1 lb of fat per day!

How do you reverse diabetes?

To reverse diabetes and melt away fat, you must control your carbohydrate choices and eat low Glycemic Index foods, while concentrating on metabolic type food ratios, exercise and balancing the adrenal, thyroid and sex hormones with the needed hormones.

To build muscle you must exercise regularly by lifting weights (temporary muscle failure) with treadmill interval training and choosing the right protein for your blood type so that when your muscles are being built, it is made from the correct protein and not an "allergic" protein.

Today, there are many supplements on the market that will aid in restoring your metabolism and they focus mainly on the adrenal glands. This is the easiest intervention in order to boost metabolism. However, some supplements have caffeine in them, which, in my medical opinion can only contribute to further adrenal burnout.

Together with eating a healthy metabolic type diet that is low in Glycemic Index and regular exercises such as bodybuilding, yoga and swimming,

---

16 ROBERTSON, W. G., PEACOCK, M., HEYBURN, P. J., HANES, F. A., RUTHERFORD, A., CLEMENTSON, E., SWAMINATHAN, R. and CLARK, P. B. (1979), Should Recurrent Calcium Oxalate Stone formers become Vegetarians?. British Journal of Urology, 51: 427–431.
17 Choi, H. K., Liu, S. and Curhan, G. (2005), Intake of purine-rich foods, protein, and dairy products and relationship to serum levels of uric acid: The Third National Health and Nutrition Examination Survey. Arthritis & Rheumatism, 52: 283–289.
18 Ibid 183.

supplements can really make one feel alive and full of vitality. Supplements that can achieve this are as follows:

- B complex vitamins 50mg
- Vitamin B 5 500-1000mg
- Vitamin B 6 20mg
- Potassium 99mg
- Chromium 200mcg
- Tyrosine 400mg
- Vitamin D 1000 i.u.'s
- Anti-oxidants ACE
- Licorice root extract (not with hypertension)
- Ginseng
- Ginger
- Adrenal glandular
- Thyroid glandular (with iodine)

What are the results of doing all this?

If you apply this information you will understand that your body has a certain type of metabolism that responds to certain foods and their ratios of carbohydrates, proteins and fats. Figuring this out will help balance your metabolism in the right way and while you are losing weight by burning fat your body will produce urine with ketones in it; this will make you feel more energized and active.

If you don't apply this information then you won't feel the energizing effects of choosing the right foods to boosts your metabolism.

Natural Hormones to consider when reversing diabetes

There are certain natural plant based hormones such as Pregnenolone and DHEA that can have a profound effect on helping to ease stress[19], re-

---

19 Pincus G, Hoagland H, Wilson CH, Fay NJ. Effects on industrial production of the administration of 3 pregnenolone to factory workers, II. *Psychosom Med.* 1945;7:347-352.

verse aging[20], help recover memory loss[21,22], lift depression[23,24], improve spinal cord recovery after injury[25], and reverse heart disease and weight issues (central to the diabetic patient[26] which in turn reverses diabetes). The focus is on the adrenal hormones and their relationship to the sex hormones and how much stress that particular person is under.

Pregnenolone & DHEA: the forgotten youth hormones

Pregnenolone is a pro-hormone, which helps with joint pain, fatigue, increases energy, improves color vision, restores memory (long-term therapy) and improves sex drive and mood in both males and females. It is also very helpful in getting people to confront challenges and deal with stress in a calmer way[27]. Pregnenolone is a steroid precursor hormone manufactured mainly in the adrenal glands, but is produced also in the liver, skin, brain, testicles, ovaries, and retina of the eyes.

Without a doubt, pregnenolone is the most impressive precursor hormone from, which nearly all of the other steroid hormones are made from; i.e. DHEA, progesterone, testosterone, the estrogens, and Cortisol

---

20   Enomoto M, Adachi H, Fukami A, Furuki K, Satoh A, Otsuka M, Kimagae S, Nanjo Y, Shigetoh Y, Imaizumi T. Serum dehydroepiandrosterone sulfate levels predict longevity in men: 27-year follow-up study in a community-based cohort (Tanushimaru study). *J Am Geriatr Soc* 2008;56:994-8.
21   Flood JF, Morley JE, Roberts E. Memory-enhancing effects in male mice of pregnenolone and steroids metabolically derived from it. *Proc Natl Acad Sci.* 1992;89:1567-1571.
22   Strous RD, Maayan R, Lapidus R, Stryjer R, Lustig M, Kotler M, Weizman A. Dehydroepiandrosterone augmentation in the management of negative, depressive, and anxiety symptoms in schizophrenia. *Arch Gen Psychiatry* 2003 Feb;60:133-41.
23   Strous RD, Maayan R, Lapidus R, Stryjer R, Lustig M, Kotler M, Weizman A. Dehydroepiandrosterone augmentation in the management of negative, depressive, and anxiety symptoms in schizophrenia. *Arch Gen Psychiatry* 2003 Feb;60:133-41.
24   Wolkowitz OM, Reus VI, Keebler A, Nelson N, Friedland M, Brizendine L, Roberts E. Double-blind treatment of major depression with dehydroepiandrosterone. *Am J Psychiatry* 1999 Apr;156(4):646-9.
25   Guth L, Zhang Z, Roberts E. Key role for pregnenolone in combination therapy that promotes recovery after spinal cord injury. *Proc Natl Acad Sci.* 1994;91/25:12308-12312.
26   Kawano H, Yasue H, Kitagawa A, et al. Dehydroepiandrosterone supplementation improves endothelial function and insulin sensitivity in men. *J Clin Endocrinol Metab* 2003;88:3190-5.
27   Pincus G, Hoagland H. Effects of administering pregnenolone on fatiguing psychomotor performance. *J Aviation Med.* 1944;15:98-115.

Dr Ray Sahelian MD[28], a bestselling author of many health books and a proactive health educator stated that;

*"I am 100 percent convinced that taking **pregnenolone** leads to changes in awareness and alertness & I notice an improved visual clarity . . . within an hour of dosing"*

I myself and most of my patients also notice improvement in color vision and memory function[29] and feel more motivated to live a better life[30] and the studies so far seem to prove this.

Dose: Many of my burnt-out patients take Pregnenolone in small amounts, 1-10mg / day, in divided doses through out the day to assist in the production of both Progesterone and DHEA. Liquid Pregnenolone is far better than capsule or tablet version, as it absorbs almost completely through the gums and tongue. The capsule or tablet version would experience stomach acids and therefore reduce its potency.

Side effects of excess pregnenolone can be acne, greasy hair, greasy skin and headaches. Simply lower the dose if this happens.

DHEA is made from a hormone called Pregnenolone, which in turn is derived from cholesterol. Pregnenolone and DHEA levels must be adequate otherwise we cannot cope with stress or ageing.

Pregnenolone and DHEA show profound anti-Cortisol (Stress hormone) activity and as such, can be an accurate measurement of how well the individual is coping with stress.

Less stress basically means a longer life. If one is *stressed* it is important to create a new lifestyle, an improved diet and to use natural hormones to rejuvenate the body and mind[31] in order to increase longevity[32].

As mentioned before, certain diseases are associated with *low* levels of

---

28   Sahelian R. The promise of pregnenolone. *Life Enhancement* 1997;36:5
29   Flood JF, Morley JE, Roberts E. Memory-enhancing effects in male mice of pregnenolone and steroids metabolically derived from it. *Proc Natl Acad Sci.* 1992;89(5):1567-1571.
30   De Wied D. Hormonal influences on motivation, learning, and memory processes. *Hosp Pract.* 1976;11(1):123-131.
31   Roberts E. Pregnenolone - from Selye to Alzheimer and a model of the pregnenolone sulfate binding site on the GABAA receptor. *Biochem Pharmacol.* 1995 Jan 6;49(1):1-16.
32   Roberts E. The importance of being dehydroepiandrosterone sulfate (in the blood of primates): a longer and healthier life? *Biochem Pharmacol.* 1999 Feb 15;57(4):329-46.

DHEA in both men and women such as cardiovascular diseases, Alzheimer's disease, depression, sleep disorders, weight gain or obesity, diabetes, hypothyroidism, lupus and cancer.

DHEA – sulphate	Conventional Range	Optimal Range	Deficient Range
Males	0.7 – 21.2 umol/L 2000–6100 ng/mL 200 – 610 ug/dl	14 4000 400	0 – 14 0 – 3000 0 - 300
Females	2.8 – 16.6 umol/L 800 – 6100 ng/ml 80- 480 ug/dl	9.7 2800 280	0 – 6.9 0 – 2000 0 - 200

DHEA goes on to make the hormones Testosterone and Estrogen. DHEA is the opposite hormone to Cortisol and has an anti-obesity effect by reducing fat cell stimulation, reduces excess insulin and has a hunger inhibiting effect.

DHEA rises with age, and peaks around 25 -30 in humans and steadily declines after that[33]; so that by the time we reach 75 years of age our DHEA levels have reduced to about 15-20% of what they were at the age of 20 years.

Too little DHEA will cause several diseases - directly related to its deficiency. And because DHEA is a key building block of Estrogen and Testosterone, DHEA has an enormous effect on Thyroid function[34] and allows the conversion of T4 into the more active thyroid hormone called T3.

Therapy

The easiest way to treat DHEA deficiencies is to use the oral route. You will want the expert advice of a functional physician when rebalancing your hormones as under-dosing and overdosing have their consequences. Here are some guidelines for therapy. Get regular hormone tests done.

---

33 Vermeulen A. Adrenal androgens and aging. In: Genazzani AR, Thijssen JH, Siiteri PK, editors. Adrenal androgens. New York: Raven Press, 1980:27-42.
34 Foldes JL, et al. Dehydroepiandrosterone sul- fate (DS), dehydroepiandrosterone (D) and "free" dehydroepiandrosterone (FD) in the plasma with thyroid diseases. Horm Metab Res 1983;15:623-624.

Women: 5 – 20mg /day 1 - 2- 3 x days

Men: 5 -30-mg/day 1- 2- 3 x days

If there is an excess of DHEA then the user might complain of greasy skin, acne, headaches, facial hair (in women) and moodiness. Reduce the dose to the bare minimum (1 drop / 1-2-3 x day) and retest levels.

DHEA Deficiency

DHEA deficiencies are associated with sleep problems and insomnia. Administration of DHEA has been clinically shown to improve Rapid Eye Movement phases (REM) associated with deep sleep and dream function. REM sleep is closely connected with dream function and memory storage[35]. Alzheimer patients usually have low levels of DHEA[36] and Pregnenolone.

DHEA improves immunity and modulates the expression of our white blood cells (T cells). DHEA protects a gland called the Thymus gland from Cortisol damage[37]. Excessive Cortisol damages this gland and DHEA stimulates and defends it. Our T cells, when dysregulated due to a lack of adequate DHEA, can cause the development of Rheumatoid Arthritis[38,39] and Lupus[40]. These diseases are characterized as an aberration in the behavior of T cells where the body starts to attack itself.

The Standard American Diet (SAD diet) has the effect of lowering the DHEA levels. Once again, the understanding is that consuming allergic foods causes increases in Cortisol, which in turn reduces the levels of DHEA

---

[35] Freiss E, Trachsel L, Guldner J, Schier T, Steiger A, Holbsboer F. DHEA administration increases rapid eye movement sleep and EEG power in the sigma frequency range. Am J Physiol 1995; 268(31):E107-E113.

[36] Bologa L, Sharma J, Roberts E. Dehydroepiand-rosterone and its sulfated derivative reduce neuronal death and enhance astrocytic differentiation in brain cell cultures. J Neuro-Sci Res 1987;17:225-234.

[37] Maes M, Holmes E, Rogers W, Pot M. Protection from glucocorticoid induced thymic involution by dehydroepiandrosterone. Life Sci 1990;46:1627-1631.

[38] Keith S. Kanik, George P. Chrousos, H. Ralph Schumacher, Marianna L. Crane, Cheryl H. Yarboro, and Ronald L. Wilder, Adrenocorticotropin, Glucocorticoid, and Androgen Secretion in Patients with New Onset Synovitis/Rheumatoid Arthritis: Relations with Indices of Inflammation, JCEM 2000 85: 1461-1466;

[39] Hedman M, Nilsson E, de la Torre B. Low sulpho-conjugated steroid hormone levels in systemic lupus erythematosus. Clin Exp Rheumatol 1989;7:583-588.

[40] Suzuki T, Suzuki N, Engleman EG, Mizushima Y, Sakane T. Low serum levels of dehydro- epiandrosterone may cause deficient IL-2 pro- duction by lymphocytes in patients with sys- temic lupus erythematosus (SLE). Clin Exp Immunol 1995;99:251-255.

via the hypo-pituitary axis. This could be a major cause of heart attacks because the SAD diet creates low DHEA, which can create increased levels of atherosclerosis and a heart attack situation[41].

DHEA levels in patients with high blood pressure[42] were typically lower than those who had normal blood pressure. Cortisol raises blood pressure by retaining the sodium levels through the mineralocorticoid pathway.

A John Hopkins University report recognized that there was a profound link between levels of DHEA and the risk of heart attacks[43]. The report recommended that DHEA could provide an accurate measurement of who would suffer from a heart attack by using DHEA levels as a marker.

DHEA is regarded as a modifiable factor in the cause of heart attacks.

DHEA studies related to the development of cancer have shown that patients with *low* levels of DHEA have greater risks of prostate cancer, gastric cancer[44], bladder cancer[45] and lung cancer[46].

In conclusion, it is important to have levels of DHEA accurately tested and monitored because the risks of developing age related degenerative disease is directly proportional to the amount of DHEA in circulation.

Maladaptation to stress causes the DHEA/Cortisol ratios to shift in a negative direction. Balance is the key and both DHEA and Cortisol are needed by the body in order to age well.

---

41   Herrington DM, Gordon GB, Achuff SC, Trejo JF, Weisman HF, Kwiterovich Jr PO, Pearson TA. Plasma dehydroepiandrosterone and dehydroepiandrosterone sulfate in patients undergoing diagnostic coronary angiography. J Am Coll Cardiol 1990;16(4):862-70.
42   Nowaczynski WF, Fragachan F, Silah J, Millette B, Genest J. Further evidence of altered adrenocortical functions in hypertension: dehydroepiandrosterone secretion rate. Can J Biochem;1968;46:1031-1038.
43   Ibid 213
44   Gordon GB, Helzlsouer KJ, Alberg AJ, Comstock GW. Serum levels of dehy- droepiandrosterone and dehydroepiandros- terone sulfate and the risk of developing gas- tric cancer. Can
45   Gordon GB, Helzlsouer KJ, Comstock GW. Serum levels of dehydroepiandrosterone and its sulfate and the risk of developing bladder cancer. Cancer Res 1991;51(5):1366-9.
46   Bhatavdekar JM, Patel DD, Chikhlikar PR, Mehta RH, Vora HH, Karelia NH, et al. Levels of circulating peptide and steroid hormones in men with lung cancer. Neoplasma 1994; 41(2):101-3.

Progesterone

In the early 1990's Dr John Lee M.D. pioneered and published articles and many books on the advantages of natural progesterone to help with menopausal symptoms, premenstrual syndrome and breast cancer.

Dr. Lee coined the phrase "natural progesterone" to differentiate real progesterone from *synthetic* progestin, because natural progesterone has such a holistic effect on the body, whereas synthetic progestins, made from petroleum such as medroxy-progesterone acetate, are recognized as a carcinogen and have an extremely narrow effect, which can cause some nasty negative estrogen based side-effects.

Unfortunately, because of the development and controlled evolution of progestins by the pharmaceutical industry, mainstream medicine does not make the important differentiation between natural progesterone and the synthetic progestins.

The pharmaceutical industry has had a strong hold over the development of progestins. Few understand that there is a *real* difference between natural progesterone and synthetic progestins[47]. Synthetic progestins, like Provera or medroxyprogesterone MPA, can create strong side effects including greater risk of heart disease, cancer, estrogen dominance, abnormal menstrual flow, fluid retention, nausea, depression and can even increase the risk of stroke.

The lack of understanding by many medical practitioners of this basic point of difference has been the source of great controversy for many years in medical fields. What's interesting about natural progesterone is that it has a beneficial effect on blood sugar regulation and helps with diabetes, where as the synthetic progestins do not help blood sugar control as progestins break down in the liver into potent estrogens.

Estrogen and progesterone, balance is the key

Estrogen, known commonly as a female hormone, is also found in men. This hormone is needed by both sexes, it has been understood that too

---

47 http://www.mercola.com/article/progesterone/cream.htm : accessed April 2012.

much estrogen in the body can cause weight gain[48], obesity[49,50], diabetes and cancer in both men and women.

ESTROGEN EFFECTS	PROGESTERONE EFFECTS
Builds up uterine lining (proliferation)	Maintains uterine lining (secretory)
Stimulates breast tissue	Protects against fibrocysts
Increases body fat	Helps use fat for energy
Salt and fluid retention	Diuretic
Depression, headache/migraine	Anti-depressant
Interferes with thyroid hormone	Facilitates thyroid hormone action
Increases blood clotting	Normalizes blood clotting
Decreases libido	Restores libido
Impairs blood sugar control	Regulates blood sugar levels
Increases risk of endometrial cancer	Protects from endometrial cancer
Increases risk of breast cancer	Probable prevention of breast cancer
Slightly restrains bone loss	Stimulates bone building
Reduces vascular tone	Propagates growth of embryo
	Precursor of corticosteroid production

(Ref: Lawley Pharmaceuticals, 2010 Australia)

Excess estrogen in men can cause prostate disorders, which ultimately can lead to an enlarged prostate[51] and prostate cancer, the 2nd greatest killer of men, and where heart disease is no.1.

Excess estrogens in women can cause lupus[52], rheumatoid and breast

---

48 M. A. KIRSCHNER, E. SAMOJLIK, M. DREJKA, E. SZMAL, G. SCHNEIDER, and N. ERTEL, Androgen-Estrogen Metabolism in Women with Upper Body *Versus* Lower Body Obesity , JCEM 1990 70: 473-479; doi:10.1210/jcem-70-2-473
49 GEORGE SCHNEIDER, MARVIN A. KIRSCHNER, RICHARD BERKOWITZ, and NORMAN H. ERTEL
Increased Estrogen Production in Obese Men
JCEM 1979 48: 633-638;
50 E. SAMOJLIK, M. A. KIRSCHNER, D. SILBER, G. SCHNEIDER, and N. H. ERTEL, Elevated Production and Metabolic Clearance Rates of Androgens in Morbidly Obese Women, JCEM 1984 59: 949-954
51 ULRICH SEPPELTCorrelation among Prostate Stroma, Plasma Estrogen Levels, and Urinary Estrogen Excretion in Patients with Benign Prostatic Hypertrophy. JCEM 1978 47: 1230-1235
52 RICHARD BUCALA, ROBERT G. LAHITA, JACK FISHMAN, and ANTHONY CERAMI
Increased Levels of 16α-Hydroxyestrone-Modified Proteins in Pregnancy and in Systemic Lupus Erythematosus

cancer[53]. Excess synthetic estrogens are the 2nd greatest killer of women in the form of cancer; and just like men, heart disease is the biggest killer[54].

Synthetic estrogens have been overused in our farm animals and in our environment for several decades since their mass introduction in society post World War II. Birth control, hormone replacement therapy, plastics, cosmetics all carry estrogens-like molecules within their structures.

There is so much estrogen and estrogen-like substances in our environment that most people will suffer from a gradual estrogen effect at some point in their lives. Women take estrogen in the form of hormone replacement therapy and birth control pills. Most consume a diet laced with estrogens and use household products that have estrogen effects within the body. Men are prone to excess estrogen and lowering of the Testosterone and as a result they become fat, have male-boobs and diabetes.

Below is a Genova lab report showing unbalanced estrogens.

Hormone	Reference Range	Reference Range
Estrone Sulfate (E1S)	2.18	0.56-2.67 ng/mL
Estrone (E1)	85	20-95 pg/mL
Estradiol (E2)	33	20-160 pg/mL
Estriol (E3)	113	<= 80 pg/mL

Estrogen must be balanced by another hormone called Progesterone.

Therefore, if a woman is prescribed estrogens long-term in the form of birth control pills or hormone replacement therapy, or eats far too many types of meat laced with estrogen derivatives, the estrogen levels will start to

---

JCEM 1985 60: 841-847
53 DANY CHALBOS, FRANÇOISE VIGNON, IAFA KEYDAR, and HENRI ROCHEFORT, Estrogens Stimulate Cell Proliferation and Induce Secretory Proteins in a Human Breast Cancer Cell Line ($T_{47}D$), JCEM 1982 55: 276-283;
54 Women's health: Preventing the top 7 threatshttp://www.mayoclinic.com/health/womens-health/WO00014

rise and become out of balance compared to the progesterone. This situation is called *estrogen dominance*. Below is a table that shows the optimal ranges required for good health.

Hormone Blood Test	Conventional Range	Optimal Range	Abnormal Range
Estradiol- women ★	0 – 528 pg/ml	352 -528	0 - 351
Progesterone- women ★	3 – 27 ng/ml	13 – 23	0 - 10
Estradiol - men	10 – 56 pg/ml	10- 25	High > 30
Progesterone- men	0.1 – 1.3 ng/ml	1.0-1.2	0 – 0.9

★21st day is the best day to test pre-menopausal (for pregnancy) women and any day for a post-menopausal woman. Estrogen levels should be measured against progesterone to see if they in balance with each other.

Progesterone		
Hormone	Reference Range	Reference Range
Progesterone	0.61	0.30-1.13 ng/mL

Diseases that are associated with Estrogen dominance are as follows:

- Weight gain – increased body fat
- Uterine fibroids
- Uterine cancer in women
- Prostate cancer in men
- Breast cancer
- PMS
- Sleep disorders
- Mood swings
- Thyroid disorders
- Auto-immune diseases

- Hypoglycemia
- Hair loss / alopecia
- Water retention
- Lupus and RA
- Chronic allergies

Also in our environment are chemicals that act like estrogens, which are called Xenoestrogens. Usually these chemicals and pesticides are laced onto vegetables and meat products. These chemicals can cause hormone balance disruptions for both men and women.

These Xenoestrogens are chemicals that can stimulate the body to become overweight and diabetic and can cause the body to store a lot of body fat. In men it can cause the development of male boobs or breasts, otherwise known as gynecomastica. Interestingly, men with high estrogen levels become fat and overweight. Women also generally have larger and larger breasts in the presence of high estrogens and pre-pubescent girls mature faster than normal girls and they reach menarche (get their first periods at an earlier age).

Our society is *riddled* with estrogens on multiple levels, from birth control to hormones in post-menopausal women as well as cattle sold for consumption, and this of course sets up an eventual decline in progesterone.

Ultimately the estrogens and the Xenoestrogens set up an imbalance within our system where the progesterone levels become too low and of course the progesterone deficiency disease will then manifest (e.g. fibroids, breast cancer, ovarian cancer, endometriosis, prostate problems, and fertility issues.)

Therapy

Relief is found in getting the body to detoxify from estrogens by eating cruciferous vegetables (broccoli, cabbage, Brussels sprouts, ramping up the liver function (milk thistle) and making sure that the blood chemistry liver enzymes (zinc & selenium) are within optimal ranges or as good as they can be. Hormonally progesterone therapy will also achieve great results because it makes up the deficient hormone, which in turn reboots the endocrine system and the organs of the body.

Only a physician must administer progesterone and/ or estrogen therapy. Prescriptions in the form of oral tablets, sub-lingual's or transdermal creams are the normal method of absorption.

To test for estrogens and progesterone I would suggest as a professional to order a comprehensive hormonal profile (progesterone, estrogens, DHEA, testosterone etc) that includes 2 Hydroxyestrone (2:OHE) and 16 alpha Hydroxyestrone (16a OHE) and estrogen metabolism ratio. The former is the good 'light' estrogen and the latter is the bad 'heavy' estrogen.

Estrogen Metabolism

Hormone	Reference Range	Reference Range
2-Hydroxyestrone	299	112-656 pg/mL
16α-Hydroxyestrone	323	213-680 pg/mL
2:16α-Hydroxy-Estrone Ratio	0.93	0.40-1.40

16aOHE is the major cause of breast cancer, rheumatoid and lupus. Making sure that the basic hormones of the estrogens (E1, E2, E3), progesterone and testosterone are balanced, whilst keeping the 16aOHE lower in concentration than the 2OHE, will keep women free from breast cancer and other auto-immune diseases. This fact also applies to men.

Low thyroid function or hypothyroidism is closely associated with low progesterone and low DHEA (vice versa).

Testosterone

As with all the hormones, testosterone declines with age and men and women over the age of thirty will have a certain degree of deficiency, namely because DHEA levels decline after the age of 25 -30 years. DHEA converts into the androgen strength and sexuality hormone called testosterone.

Commonly thought of as a male hormone, testosterone is required by both the sexes as it relates to muscle development and libidinal function. Testosterone is an anabolic hormone, which builds muscle and *reduces fat,* and which can easily be tested using a simple blood test.

Disease susceptibility in men with low testosterone sets them up for several diseases such as heart attacks, prostate cancer, high blood pressure, elevated cholesterol, blood clots, type 2 diabetes, depression, very low libido and infertility.

Disease susceptibility in women with low testosterone can cause depression, joint pain such as osteoarthritis or rheumatoid, anxiety and atherosclerosis and a very low libido .

Total Blood Testosterone	Conventional range	Optimal Range	Deficient range
Male	10-35 nmol/L 3000-10000 pg/ml 300-1000 ng/dL	24 7000 700	0 – 19 0 – 5500 0 -550
Female	0.3-1.7nmol/L 100-500 pg/ml 10-50 ng/ml	1.2 350 35	0 - 0.9 0 - 250 0 - 25
Free Testosterone			
Male	6 – 26.5 pg/ml	20-26 pg/ml	0- 15

Both sexes will typically suffer from common complaints such as low sex drive, excessive emotions and anxieties, low resistance to stress and poor muscle strength. Testosterone replacement therapy in both sexes will improve muscle function[55][56][57].

---

55 Shalender Bhasin, Thomas W. Storer, Nancy Berman, Kevin E. Yarasheski, Brenda Clevenger, Jeffrey Phillips, W. Paul Lee, Thomas J. Bunnell, and Richard Casaburi. Testosterone Replacement Increases Fat-Free Mass and Muscle Size in Hypogonadal Men. JCEM 1997 82: 407-413

56 Fred R. Sattler, Carmen Castaneda-Sceppa, Ellen F. Binder, E. Todd Schroeder, Ying Wang, Shalender Bhasin, Miwa Kawakubo, Yolanda Stewart, Kevin E. Yarasheski, Jagadish Ulloor, Patrick Colletti, Ronenn Roubenoff, and Stanley P. Azen, Testosterone and Growth Hormone Improve Body Composition and Muscle Performance in Older Men. JCEM 2009 94: 1991-2001

57 Chevon M. Rariy, Sarah J. Ratcliffe, Rachel Weinstein, Shalender Bhasin, Marc R.

NB: Testosterone therapy warrants the advice and management of a competent physician. Measuring Free Testosterone in the blood is also important as it represents a true picture of how much testosterone is available for use by the body.

In men the optimal range for free Testosterone is 20-26 pg/ml [58]. The average lab or MD will use a range of 6 – 26.5 pg/ml. This is allowing men to get unnecessarily ill as the reference range is so wide that it's hard to spot the connections between disease development and testosterone decline[59]. A low level of testosterone places every man at greater risk for virtually every age related disease. Below is a table to show the blood testosterone decline over the years[60].

Male / Age Groups	Mean
30-39	12.84
40-49	12.42
50-59	11.38
60-69	10.71
70 plus	9.5

Testosterone levels decline gradually with age in human beings this is clear from the above table[61]. The clinical significance of this decrease is debated. There is disagreement about *when* to treat aging men with testosterone replacement therapy.

The American Society of Andrology's position is that "testosterone replacement therapy in aging men is indicated when both clinical symptoms

---

Blackman, Jane A. Cauley, John Robbins, Joseph M. Zmuda, Tamara B. Harris, and Anne R. Cappola. Higher Serum Free Testosterone Concentration in Older Women Is Associated with Greater Bone Mineral Density, Lean Body Mass, and Total Fat Mass: The Cardiovascular Health Study. JCEM 2011 96: 989-996
58 Faloon W. Physician's guide: Using blood tests to safely induce weight loss. Life Extension Magazine. 2009 Jun;15(6):42-63.
59 Turhan S, Tulunay C, Güleç S, et al. The association between androgen levels and premature coronary artery disease in men. Coron Artery Dis. 2007 May;18(3):159-62.
60 http://www.lef.org/magazine/mag2010/jun2010_Startling-Low-Testosterone-Blood-Levels-in-Male-Life-Extension-Members_01.htm
61 http://www.lef.org/magazine/mag2010/jun2010_Startling-Low-Testosterone-Blood-Levels-in-Male-Life-Extension-Members_01.htm

and signs suggestive of androgen deficiency and decreased testosterone levels are present."[62]

The American Association of Clinical Endocrinologists says "Hypogonadism is defined as a free testosterone level that is below the lower limit of normal for young adult control subjects. Previously, age-related decreases in free testosterone were once accepted as normal. Currently, they are not considered normal. Patients with low-normal to subnormal range testosterone levels warrant a clinical trial of testosterone."

Using salivary measurements, the optimal ranges are as follows:

Salivary Testosterone	Optimal Range	Deficient Range	Conventional References
Morning	420	0-300	290-520 pmol/L
Midday	300	0-240	190-350 pmol/L
Afternoon	200	0-170	140-220 pmol/L
Evening	130	0-100	50-160 pmol/L

Below is an example of a patient and their recorded testosterone levels at the four points throughout the day:

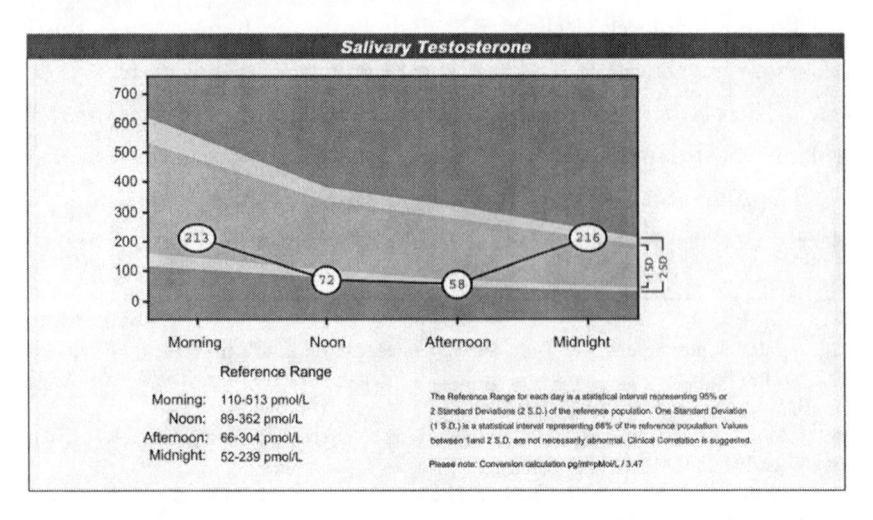

Salivary Testosterone

Morning: 213
Noon: 72
Afternoon: 58
Midnight: 216

Reference Range
Morning: 110-513 pmol/L
Noon: 89-362 pmol/L
Afternoon: 66-304 pmol/L
Midnight: 52-239 pmol/L

The Reference Range for each day is a statistical interval representing 95% or 2 Standard Deviations (2 S.D.) of the reference population. One Standard Deviation (1 S.D.) is a statistical interval representing 68% of the reference population. Values between 1 and 2 S.D. are not necessarily abnormal. Clinical Correlation is suggested.

Please note: Conversion calculation pg/ml=pMol/L / 3.47

---

62 "Testosterone replacement therapy for male aging: ASA position statement". *J. Androl.* **27** (2): 133–4. 2006.

As you can see from the above salivary testosterone numbers this patient is clearly in a low testosterone pattern. We should all be aiming for the optimal range at all points throughout the day.

It took me personally about six months to raise my *free testosterone* from 9.26 to 23.48. Testosterone therapy takes time to see results. Most results take about 3 months to see about 30-40% improvements. Monitor to see how the numbers change every three months until you are in optimal range.

Remember there are strong connections between low testosterone and the development of diabetes, heart disease and reduced lifespan. Low dose Testosterone therapy to achieve optimal health and resist disease is not the same as body-building. Body builders take in 1 month what it would need to treat a low testosterone male for 3- 5years. We are looking for optimal health, not an extreme muscular physique.

Natural Therapeutics to Boost Testosterone

Testosterone requires several co-factors in its production which are listed as follows:

- Vitamin E 400iu's
- Lipoic acid 100 mg
- Co Q10 30-120 mg
- Zinc 50 mg
- Vitamin C 1000mg
- L-arginine 500-1000 mg (avoid if there is a history of herpes)
- B complex 50mg
- DHEA 5mg-50mg (depending on blood test result and gender)
- Nettle tea (stimulate testosterone production) 1 -2 cups per day
- Bio-identical testosterone (TH 0007/Lawley Pharmaceuticals, Australia)

Testosterone, fat metabolism and increasing muscle mass are synonymous with each other and if the level of testosterone can be raised a little, the results can be quite amazing. It is a scientific fact that the majority of over-weight or obese men have lower testosterone levels, sugar issues, high estrogen and heart problems compared to slim, fit men.

Obesity is related to the risk of developing cardiovascular diseases and type 2 diabetes. One should test for testosterone to see if it is at its optimal range i.e. youthful ranges of a man around 30 years of age. As a caution men should also test their PSA levels and rule out any prostate cancer on an annual basis. However, I am of the opinion that prostate problems and prostate cancer are due to a chronic progesterone and testosterone deficiency.

Step 4

Learn about Minerals

Vegetables are the best source of vitamins from nature.

Most vegetables have a low GI value of between 15 and 30. Please note that you should always wash your vegetables well before consuming to allow the removal of dirt, dust, trace pesticides and herbicides.

Why are they good for us?

Vegetables like broccoli are generally alkaline, and if chosen wisely they can really help in the fight against cancer[1,2], obesity and diabetes[3].

Excess acidity makes insulin less effective as insulin is an alkaline substance. Generally most westerners consume way too much acidic food such as wheat, yeast, sugar, coffee, meats, pastries and these can cause the body to become overly acidic over a long time. Many medical doctors and complementary physicians believe that acidity fosters Candida infections[4]. Whether this is through the Cortisol stress response or that overly processed acidic foods carry more estrogens that favor Candida overgrowth is still yet to be answered, but the links are to be found in the clinical trenches.

---

1 Kolonel LN, Hankin JH, Whitemore AS, et al. Vegetables, fruits, legumes and prostate cancer: a multiethnic case-control study. Cancer Epidemiol Biomarkers Prev 9:795-04.
2 Keck AS, Finley JW. Cruciferous vegetables: cancer protective mechanisms of glucosinolate hydrolysis products and selenium. Integr Cancer Ther 2004; 3:5-12.
3 http://www.diabetes.org/food-and-fitness/food/what-can-i-eat/non-starchy-vegetables.html. Accessed april 2012
4 Young, Robert. Overacidity and Overgrowth of Yeast, Fungus and Moulds. Canada Consumer Health. May 1997.

With time the acidity will disrupt the key chemical processes in your organs; and eventually cause their demise and the development of pathologies such as diabetes and heart disease.

How do you prevent excess acidity?

The optimal diet is 75-80% alkaline and the rest should be acidifying foods. Using alkaline foods will help the insulin molecules to respond better. Acidity in the body weakens insulin and the reverse is also true, that alkaline bodies have stronger insulin function.

Alkalizing Foods:

- Avocado
- Sweet potato,
- Cucumber
- Celery
- Spinach
- Edema me
- Yam
- Cassava
- Cabbage
- Carrots
- Lemon
- Lime
- Broccoli
- Parsnips
- Asparagus
- Onions
- Okra
- Olives
- Tomatoes
- Lettuce
- Chives
- Artichoke
- Fresh coconut water
- Cilantro / coriander
- Vegetable juices
- Ginger
- Pumpkin
- Garlic
- Radishes
- Endive
- Leeks
- Squash
- Watercress
- Cauliflower
- Almonds
- Dandelion root
- Burdock root

Alkalizing Minerals – below are listed the alkalizing minerals with their pH value needed for proper organ and cell function.

- Potassium 14
- Sodium 14
- Calcium 12
- Chlorine 11.7
- Magnesium 10

Acidifying Foods – of course acidic food items should be eaten in small to moderate amounts so that it balances the 75-80% alkalizing foods.

- Beef
- Lamb
- Turkey
- Chicken
- Shellfish
- Tuna
- Cheese
- Eggs
- Coffee
- Tea
- Chocolate
- White sugar
- Wheat
- Milk
- Ice cream
- Bread
- Soft drinks
- Anything pickled such as gherkins, onions et

NB: when choosing the pH of your food, please refer to the Glycemic index in the appendix.

Step 5

Stress and the Side Effects

Stress is the biological term to represent the consequences of the human to respond inadequately to an emotional pressure, physical threat or spiritual fear.

The overstrain manifests a surge in adrenal hormones and over-time or great intensity, the human suffers from the decline of the adrenal hormones as the adrenals become weaker.

Chronic anxiety, constant worry, nervous tension, work pressure, the inability to relax, sleep deprivation and physical trauma all take their toll on the adrenals.

Why Beating Stress helps recover from Diabetes

If you are diabetic and fat, fatigued and depressed, this is an important chapter to understand as it will explain why you are that way.

Stress causes the body to release the hormone Cortisol, and the Cortisol levels will continue to remain high as long as the "stressor" is present[1,2]. In excess, Cortisol will cause blood sugar levels to rise and create weight gain[3] due to the fact that DHEA gets lower and as DHEA lowers, glucose destabi-

---

1   Blood GW, Blood IM, Bennett S, Simpson KC, Susman EJ. Subjective anxiety measurements and Cortisol responses in adults who stutter. J Speech and Hear Res 1994;37:760-768.
2   Opstad K. Circadian rhythm of hormones is extinguished during prolonged physical stress, sleep and energy deficiency in young men. Eur J Endocrin 1994;131:56-66.
3   Nestler JE, Clore JN, Blackard WG. Dehydroepiandrosterone: the "missing link" between hyperinsulinemia and atherosclerosis? FASEB J 1992;6(12):3073-3075.

lizes[4]. Low levels of DHEA create insulin resistance in men[5]. In women, insulin resistance (as seen in polycystic ovary syndrome) is associated with high DHEA and Cortisol.

Chronic stress over a period of time can cause peptic ulceration, IBS, [6] and tire out the pancreas's production of insulin through the damaging effects of abnormal Cortisol.

Stress also causes depression, adrenal exhaustion and lowering of the hormones and studies have shown that usually stress/depressed patients have sleep /wake cycle disorders too[7]. Over time this can lead onto chronic fatigue syndrome[8].

What you can do about it

Having the ability to modify our stress hormone responses is key to avoiding disease. Some element of feedback is necessary to gauge what the hormones are doing. Looking at Cortisol and DHEA levels as well as progesterone and testosterone plays a huge role in maintaining the overall health of the body including the pancreas and its sugar handling ability.

How can stress be avoided?

The best 'passive' way to beat stress is to be able to calm the mind and nervous system with meditation as this will lower Cortisol and help boost DHEA[9]. Clearing the mind with meditation[10] can create liberation from

---

4 Ibid 255.
5 Yamauchi A, Takei I, Nakamoto S, Ohashi N, Kitamura Y, Tokui, et. al. Hyperglycemia decreases dehyroepiandrosterone in Japanese male with impaired glucose tolerance and low insulin response. Endocr J 1996;43(3):285-290.
6 Namiki M. Aged people and stress. Jap J Geriatrics 1994;31:85-95.
7 Guéchot J, Lépine JP, Cohen C, Fiet J, Lempérière T, Dreux C . Simple laboratory test of neuroendocrine disturbance in depression: 11 p.m. saliva Cortisol. Biol Psychiat 1987; 18:1-4.
8 von Zerssen D, Doerr P, Emrich HM, Lund R, Pirke KM. Diurnal variation of mood and the Cortisol rhythm in depression and normal states of mind. Eur Arch Psychiat Neurol Sci 1987;237:36-45.
9 Linda E Carlson, Michael Speca, Kamala D Patel, Eileen Goodey, Mindfulness-based stress reduction in relation to quality of life, mood, symptoms of stress and levels of Cortisol, dehydroepiandrosterone sulfate (DHEAS) and melatonin in breast and prostate cancer outpatients, Psychoneuroendocrinology, Volume 29, Issue 4, May 2004, Pages 448-474, ISSN 0306-4530, 10.1016/S0306-4530(03)00054-4.
10 Christopher R.K. MacLean, Kenneth G. Walton, Stig R. Wenneberg, Debra K. Lev-

stress and helps to foster a mindset that is calm and relaxed. This is a do-it-yourself kind of approach to stress.

Other more 'active' ways to relax are massage, yoga, exercise, hypnosis, NLP, autosuggestion and vision boarding. Indeed the list is endless and it is important for *you* to find the *best way to relax* and recharge your nervous system and relax your tired adrenal glands.

What if you choose to ignore it?

If you don't deal with the underlying causes of stress, then you will create an adrenal overload that causes burn-out diseases such as diabetes, heart disease, cancers and repetitive headaches. Ultimately, not addressing stress will cause severe diseases and even death.

If you do beat stress then you will live a good strong life because it really helps with your adrenals, thyroid function, growth hormone and testosterone levels positively[11] . Simple!

One of the best ways to beat stress is through a supportive program designed to help the adrenal glands.

Becoming Healthier by Rebooting Your Adrenals

The adrenal glands sit on top of the kidneys within the abdomen, below the diaphragm. They are yellowish in colour and that's due to the high cholesterol content of the glands themselves. All the major hormones are made from cholesterol.

They are producers of major hormones within the body, which help to control a wide variety of functions, including mood regulation, water and salt retention (blood pressure regulation), sex drive, fertility and stress response (fight, fright or flight).

---

itsky, Joseph P. Mandarino, Rafiq Waziri, Stephen L. Hillis, Robert H. Schneider, Effects of the transcendental meditation program on adaptive mechanisms: Changes in hormone levels and responses to stress after 4 months of practice, Psychoneuroendocrinology, Volume 22, Issue 4, May 1997, Pages 277-295

11   MacLEAN, C. R. K., WALTON, K. G., WENNEBERG, S. R., LEVITSKY, D. K., MANDARINO, J. V., WAZIRI, R. and SCHNEIDER, R. H. (1994), Altered Responses of Cortisol, GH, TSH and Testosterone to Acute Stress after Four Months' Practice of Transcendental Meditation (TM). Annals of the New York Academy of Sciences, 746: 381–384

Of late, there has been a lot of change happening in world, with countries experiencing huge economic changes and political upheaval. Year on year unemployment and divorce rates have been increasing, and, therefore, the effects of stress are mounting up. The increasing stress levels that most people face, are then aggravated by the toxic environment, where the nutrition quality is totally compromised with processed foods.

Stress eating is pandemic in the USA, because eating large amounts of processed food causes a temporary rise in the feel good hormone Serotonin. This then creates an addiction to the food as a method of dealing with the chronic stress. However, the over-eating of processed food causes people to put on weight. As people gain weight this becomes another stress factor and so a vicious eating cycle is created, whereby stress leads to over-eating, which in turn leads to more stress. On top of this, body embarrassment and feelings of longing to be invisible can torture overweight individuals.

These stressful thoughts create more Cortisol, the hormone that causes *more insulin* issues. Mediation and mindfulness helps to combat the forces of stress[12].

When stressed, one of the key ways to balance it is to eat well; however, human laziness and despondency will cause people to mostly "not feel like eating healthy". Food choices are usually poor because people want to eat conveniently (because they have very little time) and also look simply for a "quick-fix" when they are feeling stressed.

Stress and exhaustion [13] can negatively affect all tissues and organs in the body. Below is a list of the diseases related to stress that I have treated in my clinic. The common denominator is the abnormal Cortisol levels and the weakening of the adrenal glands.

---

12 Ratree Sudsuang, Vilai Chentanez, Kongdej Veluvan, Effect of buddhist meditation on serum Cortisol and total protein levels, blood pressure, pulse rate, lung volume and reaction time, Physiology & Behavior, Volume 50, Issue 3, September 1991, Pages 543-548, ISSN 0031-9384, 10.1016/0031-9384(91)90543-W

13 Beishuizen, Albertus; Thijs, Lambertus G. The immunoneuroendocrine axis in critical illness: beneficial adaptation or neuroendocrine exhaustion?Current Opinion in Critical Care: December 2004 - Volume 10 - Issue 6 - pp 461-467

- Fatigue
- Diabetes
- Ulcers
- Gastric reflux and nausea
- IBS
- Asthma
- Depression
- Insomnia
- Headaches
- Low back pain
- Heart disease
- Rheumatoid arthritis
- Lupus
- Infertility
- Cancer
- Multiple sclerosis
- Ulcerative colitis
- Binge eating
- Hypoadrenia
- Hypothyroidism
- Addison's disease
- Cushing's syndrome

Progression of Stages in Adrenal Exhaustion

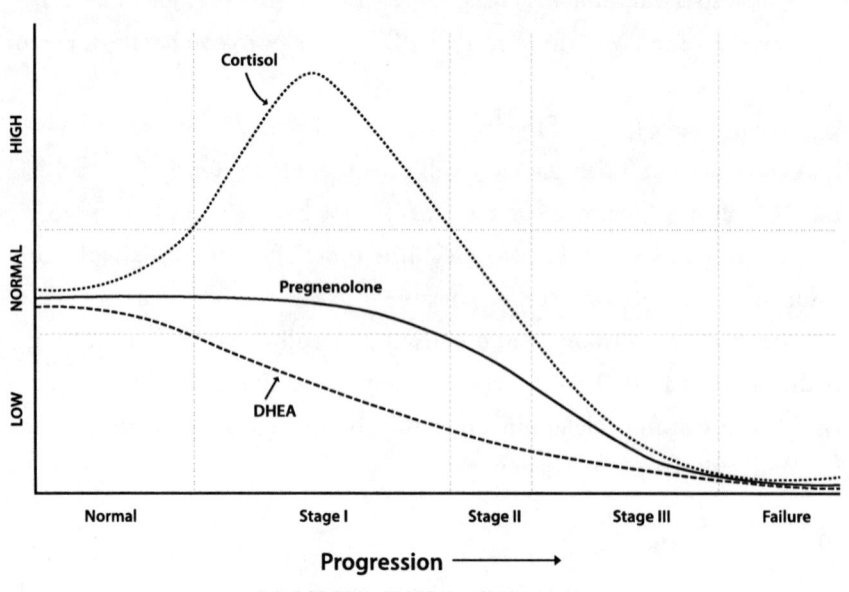

TIME OF EACH STAGE IS HIGHLY VARIABLE

There are three stages of the adrenal response and they are listed as follows[14]:

Alarm response: the first stage - as the stressor is identified, the body

---

14 Dr. Dan Kalish DC, Adrenal fatigue, Functional Medicine Training manual 2011, USA

produces adrenaline to affect the fight, fright or flight response. Cortisol is also produced.

Fatigue or Resistance response: the second stage – the stressor continues, and the body starts to tire from the persistent output of adrenal hormones. The levels of hormones start to decline with noticeable negative effects on the human body.

Burn-out & Exhaustion: is the final stage[15] - the body's resources are depleted to a point where physically the human is totally exhausted and the immune system starts to fail.

Some of the symptoms of stress are eczema, headaches, weight-gain, irritability, anger issues, diabetes, osteoporosis, cardiovascular symptoms, autoimmune disease, chronic fatigue, Alzheimer's and cancer.

Cortisol dysregulation can cause several problems, which are usually addressed by MD's only through the symptomatic medication when really the adrenals need to be tested and supported where needed with the appropriate natural hormones.

Testing the Adrenals

When testing the adrenals one has to be in mind that viral infections, allergies (wheat, gluten intolerance), mold and fungi (mycotoxins), chronic dental problems, the psychological stressors such as work issues and money issues *can all* take their toll on the adrenals.

As such, treating the adrenals requires a holistic approach. Anything less will compromise the success of the adrenal recovery program.

Make a plan and recover your health by getting regular feedback as to how well the adrenals are responding to therapy.

The basic test for testing the adrenals is called the Adrenal Cortex Stress Profile from Genova Labs, USA. The test is designed to look at two things:

1. The Cortisol rhythm during the course of the day from am to pm, and
2. The body's DHEA levels.

---

[15] Liisa Keltikangas-jävvinen· Katri Räkkönen & Herman Adlercreutz. Response of the pituitary-adrenal axis in terms of type a behaviour, hostility and vital exhaustion in healthy middle-aged men. Psychology & Health Volume 12, Issue 4, 1997

To put it simply, Cortisol is a stress hormone and DHEA is a youth hormone.

In Summary

DHEA levels are important to assess because DHEA has an anti-obesity effect. It encourages weight loss whereas Cortisol encourages weight gain or anorexia. High Cortisol levels and low levels of DHEA will cause an adverse effect on glucose/ insulin regulation and thyroid function (hypothyroidism), which in turn will slow down the metabolism.

My professional choice for testing the adrenals is performed by Genova Labs in North Carolina USA. The test is easy as it based on four saliva samples taken throughout the day.

By looking closely at this rhythm one can gauge how the body is responding to the daily stressors. One key feature to recovery is to balance the Cortisol and DHEA levels with supplements, adequate sleep (getting to bed between 9 and 10 pm) and leisure activity. Practicing relaxation is key.

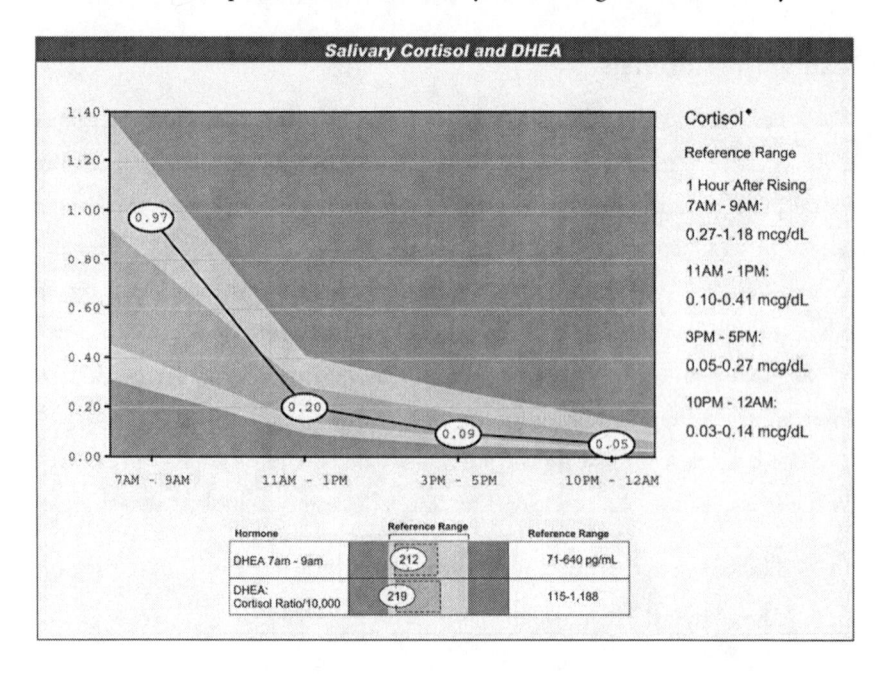

Salivary Cortisol and DHEA

Cortisol*

Reference Range

1 Hour After Rising
7AM - 9AM:
0.27-1.18 mcg/dL

11AM - 1PM:
0.10-0.41 mcg/dL

3PM - 5PM:
0.05-0.27 mcg/dL

10PM - 12AM:
0.03-0.14 mcg/dL

Values: 7AM-9AM: 0.97; 11AM-1PM: 0.20; 3PM-5PM: 0.09; 10PM-12AM: 0.05

Hormone	Reference Range	Reference Range
DHEA 7am - 9am	212	71-640 pg/mL
DHEA: Cortisol Ratio/10,000	219	115-1,188

Cortisol stress, allergies, and the Weight-gain link

When people consume unknown allergies on a daily or weekly basis the actual consumption of an allergic food (that is usually processed) will cause a stress response[16] to the body, which in turn will cause the release of Cortisol[17]. This Cortisol release upsets the regulation of sugars because "stress" causes the body to release more sugar to the muscles in response to the flight, fright or fight response.

As mentioned before, diseases associated with Cortisol dysfunction are as follows: ear, nose and throat allergies[18], food allergies, asthma[19], infections, obesity[20], schizophrenia, osteoporosis, anxiety, depression, chronic fatigue, diabetes, anorexia, cardiovascular diseases and cancer.

Eating foods that are healthy such as the Mediterranean diet succeeds in reducing the stress response[21]. Green leafy veggies and good healthy carbs, fats and proteins ensure a more robust immune system[22]. However, even within any diet system, some patients will be allergic to certain foods and IgE and IgG tests will confirm that.

As blood sugar levels repeatedly rise and fall, like a rollercoaster, the pancreas will grow tired and its ability to handle sugars goes into decline.

This sets the stage for diabetes and weight-gain.

Allergies (antigens) create anti-bodies within the blood. Antibodies are the body's response to allergies or antigens so it can recognize the difference between self and non-self.

During this process of anti-body creation, the body also makes reac-

---

16   Buske-Kirschbaum A. Cortisol responses to stress in allergic children: interaction with the immune response. Neuroimmunomodulation. 2009;16(5):325-32.
17   Stenius F, Borres M, Bottai M, et al. Salivary Cortisol levels and allergy in children: the ALADDIN birth cohort. J Allergy Clin Immunol. 2011 Dec;128(6):1335-9.
18   Chatzi L, Torrent M, Romieu I, et al. Diet, wheeze, and atopy in school children in Menorca, Spain. Pediatr Allergy Immunol. 2007 Sep;18(6):480-5.
19   Fitzpatrick S, Joks R, Silverberg JI. Obesity is associated with increased asthma severity and exacerbations, and increased serum immunoglobulin E in inner-city adults. Clin Exp Allergy. 2011 Sep 21.
20   Ibid 267.
21   Chatzi L, Torrent M, Romieu I, et al. Diet, wheeze, and atopy in school children in Menorca, Spain. Pediatr Allergy Immunol. 2007 Sep;18(6):480-5.
22   Chatzi L, Kogevinas M. . Prenatal and childhood Mediterranean diet, and the development of asthma and allergies in children. Public Health Nutr. 2009 Sep;12(9A):1629-34.

tive chemical substances such as histamines, cytokines, lymphokines and interferon. These substances act like hormones and create dramatic effects on physiology, which can have profound effects on the human nervous system, glandular systems of the thyroid, adrenals and immune system potentially knocking off normal function. IgE or immediate allergy sensitization was more common in those children with vitamin D deficiency[23]. Vitamin D is a key player in immune function.

As early as 1980's researchers and scientists were recognizing that allergic food and environmental factors[24] had been connected to a wide range of medical conditions from mild symptoms of gastric reflux to very serious diseases such as heart diseases and cancer[25]. Drugs, cosmetics and perfumes as well as certain toiletries and plastics are just as hazardous as pesticides in some individuals[26].

Allergies have also been openly associated with migraines, depression, arthritis, chronic fatigue and immune-deficiency syndrome.

Testing for Allergies

There are many advanced diagnostic labs that can perform detailed allergy screening. The method that we employ here at our clinic is based on discovering both immediate allergies using an IgE marker and delayed allergy marker using IgG.

IgE mediated responses are histamine related and when a medical practitioner encounters a suspected allergy in a patient, anti-histamines are usually prescribed. There is a large amount of medical research that supports such a strategy; however, my opinion is to *find out what the offending allergy is*, by screening the IgE antibodies carefully to understand the immediate allergy and subsequently to avoid it.

Asthma, hives and eczema are mostly IgE mediated allergy responses.

---

23   The Journal of Allergy and Clinical Immunology. Volume 127, Issue 5 , Pages 1195-1202, May 2011
24   Randolph, Theron G., Moss, Ralph W., An alternative approach to allergies: The new field of clinical ecology unravels the environmental causes of mental and physical ills. Lippincott & Crowell, (New York), 1980 Chp 4. Pg 71
25   Jerome O. Nriagu,, A Silent Epidemic of Environmental Metal Poisoning? *Environmental Pollution* 50 (1988) 139-161
26   Ibid 273 Chp5, Pg 96

IgE Food Antibody Results

Grains	RESULT kU/L	CLASS		Nuts	RESULT kU/L	CLASS
Buckwheat	0.89	II		Almond	0.24	0/1
Corn	16.31	V		Brazil Nut	<0.24	0/1
Oat	<0.24	0/1		Coconut	0.4	II
Rice	<0.24	0/1		Hazelnut	<0.24	0/1
Sesame	<0.24	0/1		Peanut	98.36	VI
Soybean	<0.24	0/1		**Seafood**		
Wheat	1.3	III		Blue Mussel	26.12	VI
Dairy				Codfish	3.89	III
Egg White	0.26	I		Salmon	<0.24	0/1
Cow's Milk	<0.24	0/1		Shrimp	3.9	III
				Tuna	<0.24	0/1

IgG Food Antibody Results

Dairy		Vegetables		Fish/Shellfish		Nuts and Grains	
Casein	0	Alfalfa	VL	Clam	0	Almond	VL
Cheddar cheese	VL	Asparagus	0	Cod	0	Buckwheat	0
Cottage cheese	VL	Avocado	3+	Crab	VL	Corn	3+
Cow's milk	VL	Beets	VL	Lobster	1+	Corn gluten	1+
Goat's milk	VL	Broccoli	VL	Oyster	0	Gluten	0
Lactalbumin	0	Cabbage	3+	Red snapper	0	Kidney bean	0
Yogurt	VL	Carrot	3+	Salmon	0	Lentil	0
Fruits		Celery	3+	Sardine	0	Lima bean	0
Apple	0	Cucumber	0	Shrimp	0	Oat	1+
Apricot	0	Garlic	1+	Sole	0	Peanut	0
Banana	0	Green Pepper	VL	Trout	0	Pecan	3+
Blueberry	VL	Lettuce	VL	Tuna	0	Pinto bean	0
Cranberry	0	Mushroom	1+	**Poultry/Meats**		Rice	VL
Grape	1+	Olive	VL	Beef	0	Rye	0
Grapefruit	1+	Onion	VL	Chicken	0	Sesame	1+
Lemon	0	Pea	VL	Egg white	0	Soy	0
Orange	0	Potato, sweet	VL	Egg yolk	VL	Sunflower seed	0
Papaya	0	Potato, white	VL	Lamb	0	Walnut	VL
Peach	VL	Spinach	1+	Pork	0	Wheat	1+
Pear	0	String bean	1+	Turkey	0	**Miscellaneous**	
Pineapple	0	Tomato	VL			Yeast	1+
Plum	VL	Zucchini	VL			Cane sugar	1+
Raspberry	VL					Chocolate	VL
Strawberry	VL					Coffee	VL
						Honey	0

Total IgE: Outside 298.0, Reference Range <=87.0 IU/mL

The patient must find out what substance they are allergic to rather than just treat the symptoms.

IgG mediated responses are delayed responses and involve a reaction within the cells. The antigen binds to the cell and this activates an immune response against the cell.

For example, let's imagine a patient who belongs to either the B or AB blood groups and who is therefore allergic to shrimp or chicken. On Sunday they visit the family for a shrimp /chicken dinner. They feel fine the next day and even the next; however, on Wednesday they suddenly develop an allergic response, such as acid reflux or a migraine.

They go to their doctor for assistance, but unfortunately their doctor, like most MD's, fails to check for IgG responses (as most only look at IgE) and so does not actually help our patient understand where the problem comes from.

Despite it being common practice for MD's not to check for IgG responses, medical literature supports the fact that 80% of allergy responses are IgG or delayed responses.

If the patient doesn't find out what the delayed allergies are, then once again the adrenals become stressed (Cortisol) and this has the domino-effect of hurting the pancreas (insulin resistance), setting the patient up for weight gain (Estrogen) and immune problems that may in turn create heart disease or, even worse, cancer.

Stress can adversely cause the glucose and insulin ratio to be profoundly upset with the ultimate effect of slowing down the metabolism. Cortisol stimulates the deposition of fat, the accelerated breakdown of muscles and joints, and induces sleeping problems such as insomnia.

The question is: what are the allergies that are making you fat? Ask your holistic minded physician to order a full 120 foods and inhalants panel for IgE and IgG. Follow the process and avoid eating those foods and environments. My preferred lab is a Genova Diagnostic lab in North Carolina, USA. I have found that they have been very accurate and reliable over the 15 years that I have been using them.

Your physician will need to take a blood sample from you in order to process the test. Understanding what substances you are allergic to will help you make tremendous health improvements and step up your metabolism for the better; which will enable you to look better and live longer!

Beating Stress with Meditation and Contemplation

Meditation is defined as the mental ability to empty the mind or the power to use the mind to concentrate on something in particular. The ability to ponder clearly on a specific subject of betterment will encourage your body and mind to achieve that goal. "Seeing" and "feeling" your goals within your mind during meditation helps you to develop a state of calmness that allows the universe to start preparing the circumstances of achieving that goal.

The purity of the meditation experience is dependent on having a good diet because the brain is influenced by the purity of the foods eaten.

When one eats processed or cheap foods that are full of yeast extracts, chemical and hormone residues, the overall effect is to ruin one's health. More so, it will ruin the quality of your thinking. Your ability to think clearly and to be sensitive to the little clues of the universe unfolding is dependent on you having an awareness developed through meditation and contemplation.

If you had to name the hormone that makes us happy and fulfilled its name would be Serotonin. The amount of serotonin in the body dictates whether we feel happy or sad. Serotonin as a neurotransmitter is found in three key areas. Over 80% of the serotonin is made in the guts, particularly in the colon and small intestines. Some serotonin is carried by the platelets and is used to make clots in wound formation and it is also found in the brain. Interestingly enough, as witnessed by dark-field microscopy, platelets can get their serotonin hijacked by yeast that uses the serotonin for their life cycle.

Research has shown that meditation increases serotonin levels[27] and this in turn makes us happier. As I had written in my first book *The Hidden Cure*[28]:

> *Psychological stress is clearly on the increase in modern societies and those nervous tensions are creating degenerative disease and violent societies. The more stress in our lives, the more the presence of high Cortisol.*

High Cortisol causes massive increases in blood sugar levels, and stresses the heart. Increasing levels of Cortisol can result in the overgrowth of yeast. High Cortisol can affect humans on a psychological level, and is medically known to induce depression, schizophrenia and paranoia.

Researchers at the University of Innsbruck discovered this when they found that patients taking long-term Prozac or other SSRI's (selective serotonin reuptake inhibitors) experienced less yeast infections and less cancer.[1]

---

27 Bujatti M, Riederer P J: Serotonin, noradrenalin, dopamine metabolites in transcendental meditation-technique. Neural Transm 1976; 39(3):257-67
28 L. Maas B.Sc. Ost, DI. Hom, The Hidden Cure and the 5 Laws of Perfect Health, Chp 1 pg 18, Wheatmark Press, Arizona 2009

The surplus serotonin in their systems created an anti-fungal environment. This means by actively striving for a good mood using natural dietary methods and fostering a good, healthy, robust body, one can kill cancer cells and a whole set of other degenerative diseases. The happier people are, the less the fungus grows, because serotonin, the happy hormone, has antifungal properties.

How To Meditate Simply

Several patients over the years have asked me to tell them a recipe for good meditation, and in my more than two decades of practicing meditation I have given them some simple ideas, which I will share with you now.

1. Find a quiet place that is free from any strong noises (I sometimes use ear plugs to achieve this).
2. Get into a comfortable posture, by either sitting in a chair with a straight back or, more traditionally, sit cross legged on a cushion on the floor.
3. Take a moment or two to install a relaxed mind by allowing your body to settle. Think about gratitude and thank your God for everything good in your world now and be really sincere. Your God knows when you are lying and when you are being genuine.
4. As you become more relaxed focus on the gentle movements of the breath in and out of the chest.
5. As you breathe in through the nose, count silently within your mind "1, 2, 3, 4, 5", hold the breath for 4 seconds and then release for 5 seconds gently out through the mouth.
6. During the breathing cycles, focus on your goals (becoming slimmer, fitter and healthier) Imagine eating healthy foods and exercising, while allowing the harmony of the thoughts and the harmony of the breath to meld with each other. Become one in the moment. Serotonin starts to build up at this point due to the happy images and the balanced breathing.
7. Practice this cycle of breathing meditation for approximately 10-15

minutes per day. Practice twice a day if you can, in the morning first thing and the last thing before retiring to bed.

8. As you become more proficient in it then extend the time to about 20-30minutes as is comfortable. Be comfortable in your time.

Practice meditation as you wake up first thing in the morning and the last thing at night before sleeping. In the morning I sit up on my pillow and give thanks for the coming day and imagine the good things that will happen to me.

If you do not want to meditate to control your stress levels then consider regular massage as a passive activity to induce great levels of relaxation.

Step 6

Learn about Exercise

Exercise[1] has been shown to clearly improve glucose handling, which is reflected in research showing that regular exercises can *double* your insulin sensitivity and improve your cardiovascular function[2]. This can be tested using an HBa1C test through your medical doctor or osteopath.

A certified, personal trainer will create a fitness program designed to improve muscularity and reduction in body fat. Exercise is key to improving glucose management, and the key issue here is to enjoy the exercise that you practice. I have patients who do yoga to help with their diabetes and other patients who choose running, walking or even bodybuilding – whatever you choose, perseverance and regularity is the key.

The HBa1C test shows how well you have stayed on the low GI diet and reflects the glucose handling of your body[3]. Standard reference range is <7% and this level keeps you in a pre-diabetic zone.

Optimal range is < 5.7%. As the diabetes reverses, the HBa1C will get lower and lower - ideally sitting slightly below 5.7%. **Exercise will really help that number come down closer to the optimal level.**

---

1 Tokmakidis, Savvas P: Zois, Christos E: Volaklis, Konstantinos A: Kotsa, Kaliopi, Touvra, Anna-Maria. The effects of a combined strength and aerobic exercise program on glucose control and insulin action in women with type 2 diabetes. EUROPEAN JOURNAL OF APPLIED PHYSIOLOGY
Volume 92, Numbers 4-5 (2004), 437-442
2 Daniel E Singer, David M Nathan, Keaven M Anderson, Peter W F Wilson and Jane C Evans, Association of HbA$_{1c}$ With Prevalent Cardiovascular Disease in the Original Cohort of the Framingham Heart Study. Diabetes February 1992 vol. 41 no. 2 202-208
3 Bennett, C. M., Guo, M. and Dharmage, S. C. (2007), HbA$_{1c}$ as a screening tool for detection of Type 2 diabetes: a systematic review. Diabetic Medicine, 24: 333–343.

When you follow a low GI principle with regular exercise there will be improvements in the HBa1C and you will also lose weight, lower blood pressure, improve cardiac function, improve kidney function and ultimately you will live longer and enjoy better health.

You can now feel good to be empowered with the knowledge that through good food choices, discipline with exercise, correct supplements and a positive outlook that you can reverse your diabetic diagnosis, overweight issues, hypertension or high blood pressure.

Why does this help? By creating extra blood flow through your muscles you will create a cellular need to absorb more sugar out of the blood stream.

Patients with diabetes must exercise and become more vascular. They must increase the vascularity of their muscles to help absorb more sugar to keep the muscle cells alive.

The idea is that, it will improve your overall cardio-vascular symptoms, and help break down fat and toxins from within your fat cells. As the fat cell numbers get smaller, the body regains its insulin sensitivity. This is good news for diabetes reversal. It will happen if you make it happen.

How do I get started?

Get in touch with a professional trainer in your chosen sport. Getting your fitness back requires attention to the amount, duration and overall fitness level of the sport program. Bring it on….build those muscles. Enjoy the exercise and start the path to feeling great again. The most surprising myth that I have learnt over the years of training that I have done in the gym, (24 + years) is the idea that people need to push the workout routines *for hours* to lose weight. This is simply not true.

From all my osteopathic studies, research and experience I have learnt that to lose weight and burn fat **one needs to exercise regularly two or *maybe* three times a week.** I have also learnt that whole body movements using strength training techniques[4] encourage greater muscularity, weight loss and fat burn[5].

---

4   Rooney, Herbert & Balhave (1994) *Fatigue contributes to the strength training stimulus,* Medicine and Science in Sports and Exercises, 26, 1160-1164, School of Physiotherapy, Univ. of Sydney, Australia

5   Tokmakidis, Savvas P: Zois, Christos E: Volaklis, Konstantinos A: Kotsa, Kaliopi, Tou-

The traditional approach to strength training is with using free weights - dumbbells and barbells are the usual choice, and have been time tested by body builders. They allow the body to increase the size of the muscles and, therefore, burn fat.

Objective: Choosing the correct weight is key.

For example, if I choose a weight for a set of dumbbell curls I will use a weight that I can easily curl to about the 7th rep and then the 8th rep becomes harder, the 9th is even harder and the 10th is so difficult that I can almost not complete the set, but I can just about do it and that's the limit. If you can't do the set, make sure you have a spotter or training partner who will assist you to get through the set.

Technique is everything so methodical slow movements with full concentration are required to get the maximum benefit. Take at least three, four, or even five seconds for each maneuver. Become slow and graceful up until the end of the set until you start to growl, and grunt and sweat starts to pour down your face. Injuries are to be avoided by choosing the right weight or resistance band and resting in between the sessions. If done properly the muscles will grow and the flab will melt away.

The quick and ideal workout would be as follows:

Warm-up and get the blood moving

Bicycle 10-15 minutes, mix up the speeds and create variety
Or Treadmill 10 - 15 minutes walking, running intervals b/w 4 – 6 mph
Or Nordic track 10 -15 minutes; mix up the speeds and create variety

Muscle Building – Less is more

Biceps curl (wrist rotations) .... 1 set of 6, 7 or 8-10 reps
Triceps extension .... 1 set of 6, 7 or 8-10 reps
Shoulder / military press .... 1 set of 6, 7 or 8-10 reps
Chest bench press/ push ups .... 1 set of 6, 7 or 8-10 reps
Back/ lat pull downs or seated rowing............ 1 set of 6, 7 or 8-10 reps

---

vra, Anna-Maria. The effects of a combined strength and aerobic exercise program on glucose control and insulin action in women with type 2 diabetes. EUROPEAN JOURNAL OF APPLIED PHYSIOLOGY, Volume 92, Numbers 4-5 (2004), 437-442

Leg squats .... 1 set of 6, 7 or 8-10 reps
Leg lunges .... 1 set of 8-10 reps
Calf raises .... 1 set of 8-10 reps

Abdominals- developing your Core!

Lying down Crunches .... 3 sets of 10 reps
Lying down Reverse Crunches .... 3 sets of 10 reps
Hanging Lateral Crunches .... 3 sets of 10 reps
Standing Lateral crunches .... 3 sets of 10 reps
Standing cross-over crunches .... 3 sets of 10 reps

Cool Down with Yoga

Yoga stretches 3 x sun salutations – on the following days Yoga is a great way to ease up the muscles from an intense workout such as the one above. Keeping your muscles stretched out post work-out helps repair muscles faster and makes them stronger. As your muscles get stronger you are regaining your youth!

Breathing cycles are important in this protocol and the breath movement is indicated:

1. While standing, stretch up to the sky with your arms (breath in).
2. Then swoop down with your arms and touch your toes, like a hamstring stretch (breath out).
3. Leave your palms on the ground and stretch one leg all the way back behind you so that the toes are touching the ground (breath in).
4. While keeping the palms on the ground, now stretch your other leg to join the first leg. Looks like a push up with straight arms (breathe out).
5. In the same push up position, make a bridge with your body (breath in).
6. In the same push up position again with straight arms, get your chin and chest to touch the floor while leaving your backside in the air, then flatten out your whole body on the floor while keeping your hands by your shoulders (breath out).

7. Go into a cobra position; lying flat push up from your arms. (Breath in) Arching your entire back with only straight arms enjoy the extension. Lean your head and neck also in extension, open your mouth and stick your tongue out as far as you can and hold for a few seconds then close your mouth (breath in and out).

8. Go back into the push up position and with arms extended bring one leg /foot up next to your hands, while leaving the other leg in a stretched position (breath in).

9. Now place both feet up by your hands. You should be back into a bilateral hamstring stretch, palms on the floor (breath out).

10. Now stretch up to the sky with your arms (breath in).

11. Now drink some water and give thanks to life and love and for being healthy.

What if you exercise?

If you exercise you will get fitter and help raise your testosterone naturally, thereby improving fat metabolism and diabetes. If your testosterone is sub-optimal then taking low doses of natural Testosterone will improve your work outs and sex drive tremendously.

If you *don't* exercise then you will suffer the effects of less energy, a potbelly, muscle laxity, joint pains and increasing cardio-vascular problems and to top it all off a low sex drive.

Step 7

The Ultimate Goal—Stabilize the Blood Glucose and Insulin Levels

If insulin is present in high concentrations in the blood and the pancreas is dysregulated consistently, then the ability of the body to control sugar levels and lose fat is impeded[1]. In obese people fasting, insulin levels as well as fasting blood sugar are usually high in insulin and must be brought under control in order to achieve any real weight loss.

When patients start achieving optimal glucose levels within the blood, the body then has the ability to burn fat. This is the primary goal to stabilize glucose and insulin levels. If insulin is in the blood, fat cannot be burnt as energy. Patients who are overweight must treat themselves as if they are diabetic and work towards constantly achieving a good, balanced blood sugar level. One key blood test that will demonstrate this is the HbA1C[2].

Testing Stability with Hemoglobin A1C (HbA1C)

The red blood cell has a life span of about four months or 120 days. And glucose combines with hemoglobin to form a substance called glycohemoglobin. The quantity of glycohemoglobin formed is in direct proportion to the amount of glucose within the blood during that 120-day lifespan. This process is called "glycosylation".

---

[1] Goldstein, D. E.; Peth, S. B.; England, J. D.; Hess, R. L.; Costa, J. Da. Effects of acute changes in blood glucose on HbA1C. Diabetes 1980 Vol. 29 No. 8 pp. 623-628

[2] S M Marshall and J H Barth. Standardization of HbA_{1c} measurements: a consensus statement. Ann Clin Biochem January 2000 37:45—46

If the patient has had too many sugars during that timeline the amount of HbA1c increases and is irreversible. In summary, if the blood glucose level is consistently elevated then the patient's ability to recover from diabetes[3] and obesity is poor. However, if the HbA1c changes and comes into optimal ranges then the patient has a very good chance of losing weight effectively.

The HbA1C test is a great way to check up on how patients are controlling their blood sugars. Research has clearly shown that the closer one can get to optimal HbA1C levels, the better the outcomes; and of course these patients avoid the complications associated with diabetes and obesity.

Fasting blood glucose levels are also very important, as these will express how well the individual is doing on a daily basis. Steady effort in the right direction will pay huge weight-loss rewards and ultimately improve the life and longevity of the patient.

Glucose Test	Conventional ranges	Optimal Ranges
HbA1C	< 7%	4.1 -5.5%
Blood glucose	65-115 mg/dl	80-90 mg/dl

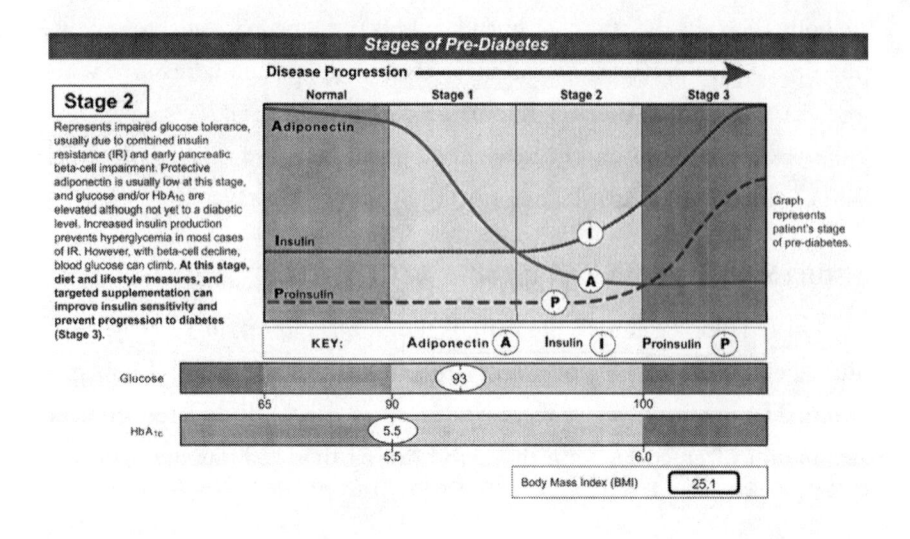

Stages of Pre-Diabetes

Stage 2

Represents impaired glucose tolerance, usually due to combined insulin resistance (IR) and early pancreatic beta-cell impairment. Protective adiponectin is usually low at this stage, and glucose and/or HbA1c are elevated although not yet to a diabetic level. Increased insulin production prevents hyperglycemia in most cases of IR. However, with beta-cell decline, blood glucose can climb. At this stage, diet and lifestyle measures, and targeted supplementation can improve insulin sensitivity and prevent progression to diabetes (Stage 3).

Graph represents patient's stage of pre-diabetes.

KEY: Adiponectin (A) Insulin (I) Proinsulin (P)

Glucose: 65, 90, 93, 100
HbA1c: 5.5, 5.5, 6.0
Body Mass Index (BMI): 25.1

---

3 Professor Eric S Kilpatrick, Department of Clinical Biochemistry. Haemoglobin A1c in the diagnosis and monitoring of diabetes mellitus. J. Clin. Pathol. September 2008 61:977—982

The above test sample shows the trending of a patient's pattern of HbA1c who is diagnosed as being Stage 2 prediabetic. As the patient continues with diet and other structured, natural therapies, the feedback testing will show the gradual recovery of normal pancreatic function.

Adiponectin[4] is a protein hormone that modulates a number of metabolic processes, including glucose regulation and fatty acid catabolism. Adiponectin is exclusively secreted from adipose tissue into the bloodstream and is very abundant in plasma relative to many hormones. Levels of the hormone are inversely correlated with body fat percentage in adults. The hormone plays a role in the suppression of the metabolic derangements that may result in type 2 diabetes, obesity, atherosclerosis, non-alcoholic fatty liver disease (NAFLD) and an independent risk factor for metabolic syndrome. Adiponectin in combination with leptin has been shown to completely reverse insulin resistance in mice.

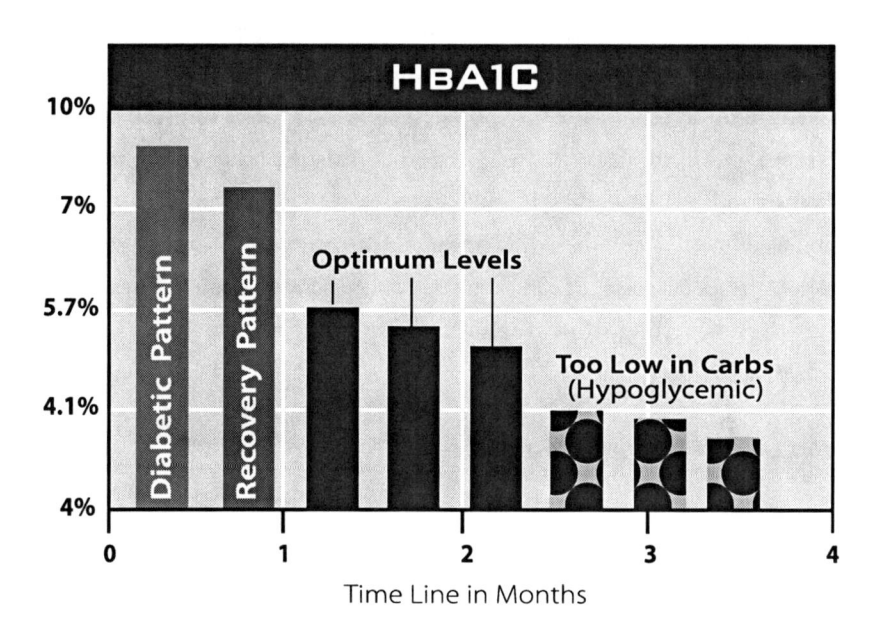

HbA1C

Diabetic Pattern: 10%
Recovery Pattern: 7%
Optimum Levels: 5.7%
Too Low in Carbs (Hypoglycemic): 4.1%
4%

Time Line in Months (0-4)

A Word about Glucagon

Glucagon is the name of the hormone that deals with carbohydrate metabolism when glucose levels in the blood start to fall. Glucagon causes the

---
4   Wikipedia- http://en.wikipedia.org/wiki/Adiponectin . Accessed April 2012

liver to release glycogen (stored glucose) and converts it into glucose and gently releases it into the blood to maintain the blood glucose levels. Glucagon is a catabolic 'fat-burning' hormone. It is the reverse of the fat causing hormone insulin.

When you eat proteins regularly they help to release glucagon. The action of glucagon is the opposite of insulin. By regulating insulin better with improved food choices, the body will start to produce more glucagon. Balancing insulin is key to weight loss. Glucagon helps the body to break down stored glycogen and fat. Increased glucagon release is stimulated by the sympathetic nervous system, that portion of the nervous system that is used during the day when one is stimulated.

Being active through a variety of exercises such as walking, running, swimming (colder water) and gym work outs all help to create a balance between insulin and glucagon. Getting excited about things helps with weight loss, so encourage more enthusiasm about the workouts that you are going to do and this will help you to become slimmer.

Glucagon is responsible for lipolysis; this is the process of breaking down fat stored within the fat cells. When this happens the body goes into a state of ketosis and ketone bodies are then excreted into the urine. When you are losing weight ketone bodies will appear in the urine, confirming weight loss through the breakdown of fat. Ketones can be tested in a lab through urinalysis. Ketone testing strips are also available on the market as well for home use feedback.

Symptoms of Hyperglycemia

1. Excessive hunger
2. Frequent thirst
3. Frequent urination
4. Obesity
5. Poor wound healing
6. Increased risk of cardiovascular diseases
7. Fatty liver changes

Symptoms of Hypoglycemia

1. Strong craving for sugars and sweets
2. Crave coffee or chocolates in the afternoon
3. Sleepy in the afternoon
4. Eating relives tiredness
5. Headaches if meals are skipped or delayed
6. Low blood pressure
7. Hyperinsulinism causes depression of blood glucose

If one balances the blood sugars scientifically using the low GI diet strategy at each plate/meal/snack of food that you eat, one can avoid all the symptoms of hyper- and hypo-glycaemia for good, thereby shifting your metabolism into better direction, reversing disease, burning fat and feeling mentally way better. Simple.

Conclusion

You are able to take control of your diabetes, one week at a time, by following the seven steps in this book.

Within one week you should see your blood sugars change for the better by a certain percentage %. If you are happy with this percentage improvement, then in four to eight weeks you'll be amazed at your new health. Your new anti-diabetic lifestyle, with better food choices such as enjoying low GI carbohydrates and removing cheap, sugary, processed foods from your diet, will make you live longer and have fewer diseases!

Putting it all together

Each day make a point of learning one key lesson and applying it. Let's recap:

- Step 1 = Eat low Glycemic Index carbohydrates from now on.
- Step 2 = Choose the correct amount of protein for your blood type.
- Step 3 = Boost your metabolism with the correct **ratio** of protein fats and carbohydrates (Metabolic type diet) – use natural hormones if needed.
- Step 4 = Choose the right alkaline vegetables and vitamins.
- Step 5 = Meditate for 5-20 minutes each day and decrease your stress.
- Step 6 = Exercise regularly and build muscles.

- Step 7 = Test your fasting blood sugars daily and HbA1c at least every three months, and watch the numbers improve.

These are the seven steps that will help you to reverse your Type 2 diabetes.

Appendices

- Useful Contacts
- Glycemic Indexes of Selected Foods
- Results, Interpretation Charts, and Treatment Guides
- Healthy Recipes

Useful Contacts

For Lab testing of the adrenals, sex hormones and allergies:

Genova Diagnostic Laboratory

63 Zillicoa St Asheville, NC 28801-1074
828-253-0621
800-522-4762
Fax: 828-252-9303
Email: cs@gsdl.com
www.gsdl.com

For Ordering Pregnenolone, DHEA, Adrenal glandulars

Energetix USA

209 West Deerfield Lane Dahlonega, GA 30533
United States
800.990.7085
866.924.6350 *info@goenergetix.com*

For Ordering Bio-Identical Progesterone and Testosterone

Lawley Pharmaceuticals (quote agent no: The 0007)

61 Walcott St
Mount Lawley, WA, 6050
Australia
http://www.lawleypharm.com.au/oo-australia.html

Glycemic Indexes of Selected Foods

Below is a shopping list of foods and their Glycemic Index. Those carbohydrates above the GI of 50-60 require some insulin or pancreatic involvement, which causes storage of the sugar as fat. Whereas slow carbohydrates with a GI of between 10 and 50 will encourage better usage of energy and help balance the weight. Combining the carbohydrates with a good portion of protein and vegetables will cause the Glycemic load to slow down.

Protein - proteins must be chosen *according to blood type* theory and preferably they could be organic and free from hormones/ antibiotics.

- Beef
- Chicken
- Turkey
- Ostrich
- Cornish hens
- Eggs
- Rabbit
- Fish
- Lamb & mutton

Dairy - Consider using organic sources and follow the blood-type rules for dairy, as it is considered a protein. For example only B and AB are allowed cow's milk and O blood must use dairy sparingly.

- Butter, ghee
- Goat's cheese
- Feta cheese
- Mozzarella
- Ricotta
- Yoghurt (live acidophilus)
- Cottage cheese
- Milk (organic cows or goats)
- Milk beverages (soy and almond are good replacements)

Vegetables - most vegetables are of low GI values of between 15 and 30. Wash vegetables before consuming.

- Arugula (10)
- Artichoke (20)
- Asparagus (15)
- Avocado (10)
- Bamboo (20)
- Bok Choy (15)
- Broccoli (15)
- Brussels sprouts (15)
- Cauliflower (15)
- Courgettes (zucchini) (15)
- Celery (15)
- Chicory, endive (10)
- Chives (5-10)
- Christophene (30-35)
- Collards (20)
- Cilantro (1)
- Cucumbers (15)
- Garlic (30)
- Hearts of Palm (20)
- Kale (15-20)
- Lettuce (15)
- Okra (20)
- Olives (15)
- Onions (15)
- Parsley (5)
- Peppers (10-15)
- Squash (75)
- Pumpkin (75)
- Spinach (15)
- Tomatoes (30)
- Sundried tomatoes (35)
- Water chestnut (60)
- Watercress (10)

Carbohydrates - if one is confident that there is no yeast activity in the body then one can choose a slightly higher GI food in order to supply more glucose for the upcoming workout or training session of physical activity.

- Carrots (16-33)
- Cassava/yucca (46 -50)
- Black eyed Peas (38-52)
- Green Peas (48-50)
- Parsnips /boiled (52)
- Yam (36-50)
- Sweet potato (50-54)
- Brown rice (55)
- Baked Beans (48)
- Kidney Beans (23-52)
- Chickpeas (36-38)
- Turnips (90)

Fruits - Always wash and clean the fruit before consuming. Once again, a higher GI fruit will supply good energy for a boosted workout from the extra sugar in the system. Only eat lower GI fruits if one is sedentary after eating the fruit. Higher GI fruits require vigorous exercise to burn off the sugar and fat.

- Green apples (35-38)
- Grapes (42-46)
- Banana (52-54)
- Cherries (22)
- Pink grapefruits (25)
- Lemons (v.low)
- Limes (v.low)
- Blueberries (40-50)
- Blackberries (40-50)
- Boysenberries (40-50)
- Raspberries (40-50)
- Strawberries (40)
- Apricots (35-38)
- Pears (38)
- Plums (39)
- Peaches (40-42)
- Mangos (41-56)
- Pineapple (51)
- Honey (60)

Herbs and Other Foods - In order to ensure that there is enough variety in the diet other miscellaneous allowable food and beverage items have been listed in the interest of clarity. Herbs, spices and other natural flavorings have no calories so make sure you make the meals tasty and full of flavor. It's much more satisfying to eat a little flavorful food than large amounts of food with no flavor!

- Honey (60)
- Chocolate/cocoa >85% (unsweetened) (20)
- Xylitol / xylose sugar (7)
- Olive oil (0)
- Cassava/yucca/yucca crackers Fiber (30-35)
- Hummus (30)
- Almonds (15)
- Hazelnut (15)
- Macadamias (20-25)
- Curry (0)
- Black pepper (0)
- Tomato sauce (30)
- Cayenne (0)
- Oregano (1)
- Vanilla (0)
- Mustard (30-35)
- Paprika (0)
- Dill (0)
- Basil (0)
- Sage (0)
- Basil (0)
- Ginger (0)

- Ezekiel bread (35)

Beverages
- Almond Milk (30)
- Carrot juice (45)
- Vegetable juice (35-40)
- Apple juice (42)
- Soda water (0)
- Coconut milk (30)
- Soya Milk (30)
- Green tea (5-10)
- Organic coffee (0)

Danger Foods with High GI's - keep away from these foods, as they will just turn into fat. It is far better to avoid these foods completely.
- Corn syrup (115-120)
- Molasses (90)
- Corn flakes (85)
- Popcorn (85)
- Glucose (100)
- White sugar (75-80)
- Fried potatoes (95-100)
- Beer (100)
- Soft drinks (70)
- Doughnuts (75-90)
- Bagels (70)
- Croissants (70)
- Biscuits (70)
- French Fries (54-75)
- Watermelon (75-90)
- White bread (90)
- Brown bread (65-80)
- Wholegrain bread (65)
- Rice milk (65)
- Wheat (70-80)
- Watermelon (90-110)

Snacks - Humans benefit from snacking in small amounts in between meals as this helps to maintain optimal blood sugar levels. Snack between breakfast and lunch say around 10.30–11am and between lunch and dinner, say around 4-4.30pm. Avoid dropping your blood sugars in between meals as this upsets the adrenals and its Cortisol axis. No delaying or skipping meals.

Have your meals ON TIME! Eat every three to four hours.

Variety and moderation is key to the success of the program, as well as an open mind as you will be educating your body to a new variety of snacks.
- Yoghurt with cinnamon or vanilla essence and almond flakes (45-50).
- Homemade chocolate cassava/

yucca/yucca crackers with flaked almonds (35-40).
- Selected low GI fruits, chopped and served with some cream and xylitol (30-50).
- Celery sticks with tuna (25-30).
- Celery sticks with cheese and olives (30).
- Avocado slices topped with melted cheese (25-30).
- Guacamole dip with cassava fiber crackers.
- Cassava/yucca crackers with melted mozzarella, garlic and tomatoes (40-45).
- Cassava/yucca chocolate biscuit (50).

Results, Interpretation Charts, and Treatment Guides

Blood Chemistry 13 Panel Interpretation Chart and Treatment Guide

TEST	DEFINITON Optimal ranges	POSSIBLE CAUSES HIGH	LOW	CORRECTIVE TREATMENT
ALT	Alanine Amino Trans-ferase 10–30 U/L	Liver issues, excessive muscle breakdown or turnover	B6 deficiency, liver issues, alcoholism	Milk thistle, B vitamins, glutamine, eggs, a very healthy diet
ALB	Albumin 4.0–5.0 g/dL	Dehydration, thyroid and adrenal hypofunction	Low stomach acid, liver dysfunction, vitamin C needed	Digestive enzymes, good hygiene, egg whites, zinc, and vitamin C
ALP	Alkaline phosphatase 70–100 U/L	Biliary obstruction, liver cell damage, bone loss, growth and repair, leaky gut	Zinc deficiency, birth control pills, corticosteroids, and hormone replacement therapy	Zinc and fat digestion, enzymes, milk thistle, increase protein consumption (eggs and salmon), B vitamins, broccoli and pumpkin, asparagus, a very healthy diet

TEST	DEFINITON Optimal ranges	POSSIBLE CAUSES HIGH LOW		CORRECTIVE TREATMENT
AMY	Amylase 60–100mg/dl	Pancreatitis	Damage to amylase-producing cells in pancreas	Chromium, pancreatin enzymes, amylase enzymes, broccoli, grape juice, royal jelly B5
AST	Aspartate amino transferase 10–30 U/L	Developing congestive heart picture, cardiovascular dysfunction, acute myocardial infarction, liver issues, excessive muscle breakdown	B6 deficiency, alcoholism	B6 and B complex, COQ10 (high doses), magnesium, calcium, potassium, vitamins A, C, and E, glutamine, increase protein intake, a very healthy diet
CA ++	Calcium 9.2–10.0 mg/dL	Hyper-parathyroidism, hypothyroidism, impaired cell membrane health	Hypo-parathyroidism, Ca needed or one of its cofactors, low stomach acid, low albumin	Betaine HCl, sardines with bones, salmon, herring, liver, vitamin D, sunshine, essential fatty acids, broccoli, asparagus
GGT	Gamma Glutamyl transferase 10–30 U/L	Biliary obstruction, liver cell damage, excessive alcohol	B6 deficiency, Mg need, kidney failure	B6 and B complex, Magnesium, glutamine, eggs, carrots and avocados, a very healthy diet
CRE	Creatinine 0.8–1.1 mg/dL	Urinary tract congestion/obstruction, renal dysfunction, drugs	Muscle atrophy/nerve-muscle degeneration, MS, liver disease, need for exercise	B complex, magnesium, potassium, vitamin D, Phosphorus, broccoli and pumpkin, asparagus, check iron levels, rule out anemia, low acidity diet

Results, Interpretation Charts, and Treatment Guides

TEST	DEFINITON Optimal ranges	POSSIBLE CAUSES HIGH	POSSIBLE CAUSES LOW	CORRECTIVE TREATMENT
GLU	Glucose 80–100 mg/dL	Insulin resistance and glucose intolerance, hyperglycemia, Thiamine need, acute stress, liver congestion, obesity, Acute pancreatitis, sugar overload	Adult and juvenile diabetes mellitus and hypoglycemia, hyperinsulinism adrenal hypofunction, alcohol, liver damage, pituitary hypofunction	Chromium, magnesium, milk thistle, COQ10, essential fatty acids, lipoic acid, low-carb diet, reduce sugar consumption use xylose as a replacement
TBIL	Total bilirubin 0.2–1.0 mg/dL	Biliary stasis or obstruction, thymus dysfunction, RBC hemolysis, sugar overload	Spleen insufficiency	Fat digestive enzymes, vitamin C, mycelized A and E, zinc, glutamine (dissolves gallstones), seriously reduce sugar consumption, a very healthy diet
TP	Total protein 6.9–7.4 g/dL	dehydration	Low stomach acid, liver dysfunction, malnutrition	Water, zinc, milk thistle, digestive enzymes
BUN	Blood urea nitrogen 10–16 mg/dL	Renal disease/insufficiency, dehydration, low stomach acid, edema	Low protein diet, malabsorption, pancreatic and liver issues	Kidney extract, B complex, magnesium, potassium, calcium, digestive enzymes, milk thistle, turmeric, low acidity diet

TEST	DEFINITON Optimal ranges	POSSIBLE CAUSES HIGH LOW		CORRECTIVE TREATMENT
UA	Uric acid 3.0–5.5	Gout, yeast and fungus, atherosclerosis, rheumatoid arthritis, renal insufficiency/disease, leaky gut syndrome, diuretics	Molybdenum, copper and/or folate deficiency, pregnancy, corticosteroids, heavy metal poisoning, occupational hazards	Magnesium, sarsaparilla, B complex, folic acid and organic lithium, nettle tea, low levels = copper deficiency (use the direction of a physician) Go on the Step 1 Diet as high uric acid can be caused by yeast

Basic Metabolic Panel Plus
Interpretation Chart and Treatment Guide

TEST	DEFINITIONS	POSSIBLE CAUSES HIGH LOW		POSSIBLE TREATMENTS
CA	Calcium 9.2–10.0 mg/dL	Hyper-parathyroidism, hypothyroidism, impaired cell membrane health	Hypo-parathyroidism, Ca need or one of its cofactors, low stomach acid, low albumin,	Betaine HCl, sardines with bones, salmon, herring, liver, vitamin D, sunshine, essential fatty acids, broccoli, asparagus
CL-	Chloride 100–106 mEq/L	Metabolic acidosis, adrenal hyperfunction, dehydration, hyper-parathyroidism, excess salt consumption	Prolonged diarrhea and vomiting, renal dysfunction, over-hydration, adrenal hypofunction, constipation	Too little or too much sea salt, dehydration, adrenal support, digestive enzymes, electrolytes

Results, Interpretation Charts, and Treatment Guides

TEST	DEFINITIONS	POSSIBLE CAUSES HIGH	POSSIBLE CAUSES LOW	POSSIBLE TREATMENTS
CRE	**Creatinine** 0.8–1.1 mg/dL	Urinary tract congestion/obstruction, renal dysfunction, drugs	Muscle atrophy/nerve-muscle degeneration, MS, liver disease, need for exercise	B Complex, Magnesium, Potassium, vitamin D, phosphorus, broccoli and pumpkin, asparagus, check iron levels, rule out anemia
GLU	**Glucose** 80–100 mg/dL	Insulin resistance and glucose intolerance, hyperglycemia, thiamine need, acute stress, liver congestion, obesity, acute pancreatitis	Adult and juvenile diabetes mellitus and hypoglycemia, hyperinsulinism, adrenal hypofunction, alcohol, liver damage, pituitary hypofunction	Chromium, magnesium, milk thistle, COQ10, essential fatty acids, lipoic acid
LD	**Lactate dehydrogenase** 140–200 U/L	Liver diseases, acute viral hepatitis, cirrhosis; cardiac diseases myocardial infarction; and tissue alterations of the heart, kidney, liver and muscle. Lymphoma, cancer, leukemia	Reactive hypoglycemia, some drugs	Milk thistle, selenium, garlic, antifungals, COQ10, B complex, check thyroid function, rule out neoplasm, If viral, take anti-viral lysine, olive leaf extract and coconut oil

TEST	DEFINITIONS	POSSIBLE CAUSES HIGH LOW		POSSIBLE TREATMENTS
MG	Magnesium 2.0–2.3 mg/dL	Renal dysfunction, thyroid hypofunction, excess Mg- containing antacids, dehydration	Epilepsy, muscle spasm, adrenal hyperfunction, malabsorption	Green leafy vegetables, magnesium supplements. Support kidneys, low acidity diet
K+	Potassium 4.0–4.5 mEq/L	Adrenal hypofunction, dehydration, tissue destruction, renal failure	Adrenal hyperfunction, diuretics, essential hypertension, diarrhea	Support adrenals, reduce stress, laugh, meditate, get in touch with nature
Na+	Sodium 135–142 mEq/L	Adrenal hyperfunction, dehydration, Cushing's	Adrenal hypofunction, Addison's, edema	Support adrenals, reduce stress, laugh, meditate, get in touch with nature, DHEA therapy, licorice, ginseng
t CO2	Total carbon dioxide 25–30 mEq/L	Metabolic alkalosis, respiratory acidosis	Metabolic acidosis, respiratory alkalosis	Reduce antacids, adjust calciums, eat some acidic foods
BUN	Blood Urea nitrogen 10–16 mg/dL	Renal disease / insufficiency, dehydration, low stomach acid, edema	Low protein diet, malabsorption, pancreatic and liver issues	Kidney extract, B complex, magnesium, potassium, calcium, digestive enzymes, milk thistle, turmeric, low acidity diet

Full Lipid Panel Interpretation Chart

TESTS	DEFINITION	OPTIMAL RANGES mg/dL	HIGH	LOW
CHOL	Cholesterol	150–220	Primary hypothyroidism, adrenal cortical dysfunction, anterior pituitary hypofunction, cardiovascular disease, atherosclerosis, biliary stasis, fatty liver, early stage diabetes, multiple sclerosis	Oxidative stress and free radical activity, heavy metal/chemical overload, liver/biliary dysfunction, insufficient fat intake, vegetarian diet, thyroid hyperfunction, autoimmune processes, adrenal hyperfunction
HDL	High-density lipo-protein cholesterol	> 55	Autoimmune processes, hypothyroidism, insulin use, excess alcohol consumption	Hyperlipidemia and atherosclerosis, syndrome X, oxidative stress, heavy 7metal/chemical overload, fatty liver, lack of exercise, hyperthyroidism
TRIG	Triglycerides	70–110	Syndrome X, fatty liver, early stage insulin resistance, cardiovascular disease, atherosclerosis, poor metabolism and utilization of fats, early stage diabetes, adrenal cortical dysfunction, alcoholism	Liver dysfunction, thyroid hyperfunction, autoimmune processes, adrenal hyperfunction

TESTS	DEFINITION	OPTIMAL RANGES mg/dL	HIGH	LOW
TC/H	Total cholesterol to HDL ratio		Greater proportion of VLDL and LDL compared to HDL making up total cholesterol.	Greater amount of HDL compared to LDL and VLDL making up total cholesterol volume
LDL	Low-density lipo-protein cholesterol	< 120	Diet high in refined carbohydrates, syndrome X, atherosclerosis, hyperlipidemia, oxidative stress, fatty liver	Low levels of LDL reduce the risks for these diseases/dysfunctions
VLDL	Very low-density lipo-protein cholesterol	< 30	Coronary artery disease	Low levels of VLDL reduce the risks for coronary artery disease

Shopping List

The following is a list of healthy food recommended by The Maas Clinic as a guide. The food guide is based on the Paleolithic diet (Paleo or Stone Age Diet), the Blood Type Diet (Eat Right for Your Blood Type) as well as clinical observations. This guide has been specially prepared to serve for shopping and educational purposes only, and is not diagnostic. This special list contains catabolic (weight loss) and anabolic (weight gain) information and is also blood type specific. Please note; if your blood type is not listed next to a prticular food, do not eat it. In order to determine which foods are right for a unique individual, a food allergy test would have to be performed. The information from this test will provide an exclusive list of foods that are allowed or that should be avoided specifically for that individual.

Catabolic - foods eaten for catabolic purposes will promote weight loss by causing the body to burn calories.

Anabolic - foods eaten for anabolic purposes will promote weight gain and muscle building by retaining calories.

Meats	Blood Type	Catabolic	Anabolic
Beef	O,B,AB	• Cold cuts • Smoked Meat • Preserved Meat • Eat during the day to burn fat	• Fresh Meat • Eat during the evening to build muscle
Buffalo	O,B,AB		
Chicken	O,A		
Cornish Hen	O,A		
Duck	O,A		
Goat	O,B,AB		
Goose	O,A		
Grouse	O,A		
Guinea Hen	O,A		
Lamb	O,B,AB		
Liver	O,B		
Mutton	O,B,AB		
Ostrich	O,A		
Partridge	O,A		
Pheasant	O,A		
Quail	O,A		
Rabbit	O,B,AB		
Turkey	O,A,AB,B		

Fish	Blood Type	Catabolic	Anabolic
Abalone	O,A,AB,B	• Smoked Fish • Preserved Fish • Eat during the day to burn fat	• Fresh Fish • Eat during the evening to build muscle
Barracuda	O,A,AB,B		
Bass/Bluegill/ Sea/ Striped	O,A,AB,B		
Beluga	O,A,AB,B		
Blue Fish	O,A,AB,B		
Bull Head	O,A,AB,B		
Butterfish	O,A,AB,B		
Carp	O,A,AB,B		

Shopping List

Fish	Blood Type	Catabolic	Anabolic
Catfish	O,A,AB,B		
Chub	O,A,AB,B		
Cod/Atlantic	O,A,AB,B		
Conch	O,A		
Crab/Blue	O,A		
Croaker / Atlantic	O,A,AB,B		
Flounder Species	O,A,AB,B		
Gray (Dover) Sole Species	O,A,AB,B		
Grouper / Mixed Species	O,A,AB,B		
Haddock	O,A,AB,B		
Half Moon Fish	O,A,AB,B		
Halibut / Greenland	O,A,AB,B		
Harvest Fish	O,A,AB,B		
Herring / Atlantic	O,A,AB,B		
Lobster / Northern	O,A		
Mackerel / Atlantic	O,A,AB,B		

Dairy	Blood Type	Catabolic	Anabolic
Step One			
Butter / Without Salt	UNIVERSAL however please note that blood types "O" & "A" should use sparingly	Most cheeses are Catabolic in **SMALL** amounts during the morning	Most cheeses are anabolic in **LARGE** amouts during the evening
Mozarella Cheese			
Goat Cheese / Milk / Yogurt			
Feta Cheese			
Sour Cream			
Buttermilk / Low Fat			
Cream Cheese			
Ghee/Clarified Butter			
Step Two			
Colby Cheese			
Cottage Cheese			

Shopping List

Dairy	Blood Type	Catabolic	Anabolic
Casein (Sodium Caseinate)			
Edam Cheese			
Emmental Cheese			
Farmer Cheese			
Cheddar Cheese			
Gouda Cheese			
Heavy Cream			
Jarlsberg Cheese			
Kefir			
Milk / Cow /Non Fat/ Whole/Yogurt			
Monterey Jack Cheese			

Dairy	Blood Type	Catabolic	Anabolic
Step Two			
Paneer	UNIVERSAL however please note that blood types "O" & "A" should use sparingly	Most cheeses are Catabolic in SMALL amounts during the morning	Most cheeses are anabolic in LARGE amouts during the evening
Provolone Cheese			
Ricotta Cheese			
String Cheese			
Swiss Cheese			
Whey / Sweet / Dried			

Fruit/Fruit Juice	Blood Type	Catabolic	Anabolic
Step One			
Apples (Green) / Apple Juice	UNIVERSAL	Most fruits are catabolic in the morning	Most fruits are anabolic in the evening
Avocado			
Blackberries			
Blueberries			
Boysenberries			
Cherries/Cherry Juice			

Shopping List

Fruit/Fruit Juice	Blood Type	Catabolic	Anabolic
Coconut Meat / Milk			
Cranberries / Cranberry Juice			
Dewberries			
Elderberries			
Gooseberries			
Grapefruit / Red & White / Juice			
Lemons / Lemon Juice			
Limes / Lime Juice			
Loganberries			
Mulberries			
Pears / Pear Juice			
Pomegranates			
Raspberries			
Strawberries			
Youngberry			
Step Two			
Apples (Red) / Apple Juice	UNIVERSAL	Most fruits are catabolic in the morning	Most fruits are anabolic in the evening
Apricot/Apricot Juice			
Asian Pear			
Banana			
Breadfruit			
Canang (juan canary) melon			
Cantaloupe			
Crenshaw (cranshaw) Melon			
Currants (Red & Black)			
Dates (Domestic)			

Fruit/Fruit Juice	Blood Type	Catabolic	Anabolic
Figs (Dried)			
Grapes (American Type/Slip Skin)			
Guava / Guava Juice			
Kiwi Fruit (Chinese Gooseberries)			
Kumquats			
Litchis / Lychee			
Mango / Mango Juice			
Nectarines/Nectarine Juice			
Oranges/Orange Juice			
Papayas			
Peaches			
Persian Melon			
Persimmons (Native)			
Pineapple / Pineapple Juice			
Plantains			
Plums			
Prunes / Prune Juice			
Raisins			
Sago Palm			
Starfruit / Carambola			
Tangerines / Tangerine Juice			
Youngberry			

Nut / Seed	Blood Type	Catabolic	Anabolic
Almond (Butter, Milk, Cheese)	UNIVERSAL	Catabolic during the morning. Excellent as snacks	Anabolic during the evening
Beech Nut			
Brazil Nuts (Dried, Unblanched)			
Butternuts			
Chestnuts			
Filberts (Hazlenuts)			
Flaxseed			
Macadamia Nuts (Dry Roasted)			
Pecans / Pecan Butter			
Pine Nuts (Pignolia / Dried)			
Poppy Seed			
Pumpkin Seed / Butter			
Safflower Seed Kernals / Dried			
Sesame Seeds (Whole/Dried/ Butter/Tahini)			
Sunflower Seed (Kernals/Butter)			
Walnut (Black / English)			

Shopping List

Bean / Legume	Blood Type	Catabolic	Anabolic
All Step Two			
Adzuki Bean	O,A	Most beans are catabolic eaten in the morning	Most beans are anabolic in the evening
Black Bean	O,A		
Black Eyed Pea	O,A		
Cannellini Bean	O,A,AB,B		
Copper / Cranberry / Roman Bean	AB,B		
Fava Bean	O,A,B		
Garbanzo (Chick Pea)	O		
Green / String Bean	O,A,AB,B		
Jicama (Yam Bean)	B		
Kidney Bean / Red	B		
Lentils / Domestic / Green / Red	A,AB		
Lima Bean Large	O,B		
Mung Bean / Sprout	O,A		
Navy Bean	AB,B		
Northern Bean	O,A,AB,B		
Pinto Bean	A,AB		
Snap / String Bean / Yellow	O,A,AB,B		
Soy Bean / Soy Nut Butter	O,A,AB,B		
Soy Cheese /Flakes /Granules /Milk/ Fluid	O,A,AB		
Tamarinds	AB,B		
Tempeh	O,A,AB,B		
Tofu	O,A,AB		
White Bean	O,A,AB		

Shopping List

Beverage	Blood Type	Catabolic	Anabolic
Step One			
Coffee (Brewed/ Prepared with water)	A,AB	√ AM	√ PM
Green Tea (Prepared with water)	O,A,AB,B	√	
Tea (Brewed/ Prepared with Water)	O,A,AB,B	√	
Seltzer Water	O,A,AB,B		
Soda / Carbonated Water /Club	O,A,AB,B		
Step Two			
Grape Juice	O,A,AB,B		√
Liquor Distilled	O,A,AB,B		√

Condiment	Blood Type	Catabolic	Anabolic
Step One			
Apple / Pectin	UNIVERSAL	√	
Baking Soda			
Carrageenan		√	
Gelatin			√
Guar Gum			
Lecithin		√	
Mustard / Wheat Free / Vinegar Free			
Pickles / Dill Relish			
Sea Salt / Table		Small Amounts	
Vinegar / Cider			
Xanthum Gum			
Step Two			
Miso	UNIVERSAL		√
Tamari			√
Soy Sauce made from Soy			√

Shopping List

Sweetener	Blood Type	Catabolic	Anabolic
Step One			
Almond Extract	UNIVERSAL	√	
Erythritol		√	
Stevia		√	
Vegetable Glycerine			√
Xylitol		√	
Step Two			
Agave Syrup	UNIVERSAL		√
Honey			√
Maple Syrup			√
Molasses / Black Strap			√

Grain	Blood Type	Catabolic	Anabolic
All Step Two			
Amaranth	O,A,AB,B	√	
Barley	O,A,AB,B	√	
Buckwheat/Kasha	O,A,AB,B		
Essene (Manna) Bread	O,A,AB,B	Low GI	
Ezekiel Bread	O,A,AB,B	Low GI	
Gluten Free Bread	O,A,AB,B		
Kamut	O,A,AB,B		
Millet (Cooked)	O,A,AB,B	√	
Mung Bean Noodles	O,A		
Oats (Flour/Bran/Meal)	O,A,AB,B	Slow Cook	
Quinoa	O,A,AB,B	√	
Rice Cakes (Flour/Bran)	O,A,AB,B		√
Rice (Cream of / Cooked with water)	O,A,AB,B		
Rice Milk/ Puffed	O,A,AB,B		

Grain	Blood Type	Catabolic	Anabolic
Rice (White/ Brown / Basmati/ Wild)	O,A,AB,B		√
Soba Noodles (made with buckwheat only)	O,A,AB,B		
Sorghum	O,A,AB,B		
Soy Flour (Full-Fat/ Raw)	A,AB		√
Spelt (Flour / Products)	O,A,AB,B		√
Tapioca (Pearl / Dry)	O,A,AB,B		√
Teff	O,A,AB,B	√	

Herb /Spice	Blood Type	Catabolic	Anabolic
Acacia (Gum Arabic)	UNIVERSAL	N/A	N/A
Allspice			
Anise Seed			
Arrowroot Flour			
Basil			
Bay Leaf			
Bergamot			
Caraway Seed			
Cardamom			
Carob Flour			
Chervil			
Chili Powder			
Chives			
Chocolate / Cocoa			
Cilantro			
Cinnamon			
Cloves			
Coriander			
Cream of Tartar			

Shopping List

Herb /Spice	Blood Type	Catabolic	Anabolic
Cumin Seed			
Curry Powder			
Dill Seed			
Guarana			
Licorice Root			
Mace / Ground			
Marjoram / Dried			
Mustard / Dry / Powder			
Nutmeg			
Oregano			
Paprika			
Parsley			
Pepper / Black / Peppercorn / Fresh Ground			
Pepper / Black / White / Commercial Ground			
Pepper/Cayenne/Red Flakes/Jalapeno/Chili			
Peppermint			
Rosemary			
Saffron			
Sage / Ground			
Savory / Ground			
Spearmint			
Tarragon / Ground			
Thyme / Fresh			
Turmeric / Ground			
Vanilla Extract			
Wintergreen			

Oil	Blood Type	Catabolic	Anabolic
Almond	UNIVERSAL		√
Avocado		√	
Black Currant Seed		√	
Borage Seed			√
Coconut		√	
Cod Liver			√
Corn			√
Cotton Seed			√
Evening Primrose		√	
Flax Seed			√
Olive		√	
Safflower			√
Sesame			√
Sunflower			√
Walnut			√
Wheat Germ			√

Vegetables	Blood Type	Catabolic	Anabolic
Step One			
Agar	UNIVERSAL	Most Vegetables are catabolic in small to moderate amounts (Low GI)	Most vegetables are anabolic in large amounts (High GI)
Alfalfa Seeds / Sprouted			
Aloe			
Artichokes / Artichoke Flour			
Artichoke / Jerusalem			
Arugula			
Asparagus			
Asparagus Pea			
Bamboo Shoots			
Beet			
Beet Greens			
Bok Choy Cabbage			

Shopping List

Vegetables	Blood Type	Catabolic	Anabolic
Broccoli / Broccoli Sprouts			
Brussel Sprouts			
Cabbage / Common			
Cabbage Juice			
Capers			
Carrot			
Carrot Juice			
Cauliflower			
Celeriac			
Chicory Roots			
Collard Greens			
Cucumber			
Cucumber Juice			
Daikon Radish			
Dandelion Greens			
Eggplant (do not use if you have athritis or any other inflammatory acidic condition)			
Endive			
Escarole			
Fennel / Bulb			
Garlic			
Ginger Root			
Horseradish / Prepared			
Kale			
Kelp			
Kohlrabi			
Leeks			
Lettuce - All Types			

Shopping List

Vegetables	Blood Type	Catabolic	Anabolic
Mustard Greens			
Okra			
Olives - Black/Green/Greek/Kalamata/Spanish			
Onions			
Oyster Plant (Salsify)			
Pea/Green/Yellow			
Peppers-All varieties			
Pickle -Brine/Vinegar			
Pimento			
Radicchio			
Radish/Radish Sprouts			
Rhubarb			
Sauerkraut			
Scallions			
Seaweed			
Shallots			
Spinach			
Swiss Chard			
Taro/Tahitian			
Tomatoes / Tomato Juice			
Water Chestnuts/Chinese			
Water Cress/ Garden			
Yam			
Yucca (Cassava)			
Zucchini			

Shopping List

Vegetables	Blood Type	Catabolic	Anabolic
Step Two			
Parsnip			
Potato (Sweet/White/Red)			
Pumpkin			
Squash			
Turnips			

Eggs & Roes	Blood Type	Catabolic	Anabolic
Caviar/Black or Red	UNIVERSAL		
Chicken Egg (Scrambled, Fried, Omelette)		√ A.M	
Chicken Egg (Poached, Boiled, Soft Yolk)			√ P.M
Duck Egg (whole)			
Goose Egg (whole)			
Quail Egg (whole)			
Salmon Roe			

Healthy Recipes

Baked Goods:

1. Cassava Bread
2. Cassava Crepe
3. Pizza Crust Recipe
4. Cassava Chocolate Cookie
5. Cheese Muffins
6. Cassava Chocolate Cake
7. Cassava Yellow Cake
8. Cassava Nachos

Dressings:

1. Antifungal Salad Dressing/Gentle Liver Flush
2. Fresh Lemon & Coriander Dressing
3. Sweet Basil Dressing
4. Mixed Herb Yoghurt Dressing
5. Herby Mustard Dressing
6. Creamy Curried Dressing

Salsas & Pesto:

1. Salsa Verde
2. Mango & Avocado Salsa
3. Classic Basil Pesto

4. Rocket & Mint with Macadamia
   5. Red Pepper Pesto

Dips:

   1. Homemade Mayonnaise
   2. Guacamole
   3. Coriander Humus
   4. Tzatziki
   5. Watercress Cheese Dip
   6. Sour Cream & Chive Dip

Quick Snacks:

   1. Chocolate & Fruit Crackles
   2. Dried Fruit & Coconut Trail Mix
   3. Parmesan Chips
   4. Oven Baked Vegetable Crisps
   5. Mini Pizzava Squares
   6. Herbed Mahi-Mahi Kebabs
   7. Beef & Onion Kebabs
   8. Chicken Tikka Masala Drumsticks

Breakfast:

   1. Eggs Florentine
   2. Belgian Waffles
   3. Warm Bean Salad
   4. Green Bean & Egg Salad
   5. Tomato & Courgette Bake
   6. Omelet Wrap with Stir Fried Greens

Light Lunch Salads:

1. Salmon & Avocado Salad
2. Mediterranean Chicken Salad
3. Sesame Chicken Salad
4. Nicoise Salad
5. Roast Beef & Rocket Salad
6. Vegetable, Haloumi Salad
7. Fish Burritos

Dinner Ideas:

1. Poached Fish Cutlets with Mixed Greens Salad
2. Chermoula crusted Fish
3. Sour Fish Curry
4. Chicken in Yoghurt
5. Lamb and Spinach Curry
6. Turkey Lamb with Cranberries
7. Lemon Chicken with Greens

Sides:

1. Garbanzo Bean salad
2. Roasted Pumpkin with Sesame Seeds
3. Lady's Fingers in Spicy Tomatoes
4. Curried Cauliflower
5. Green Beans with Walnuts
6. Garlicky Brussel Sprouts
7. Sesame Seasoned Spinach

Carbohydrate Content:

1. Classic Yam Puree
2. Scalloped Sweet potato
3. Rosemary Roasted Ground Provisions
4. Cassava & Parsnip Mash
5. Pumpkin & Yam Puree
6. Fried Cassava Chips

Stocks:

1. Beef
2. Chicken
3. Fish
4. Vegetables

Soups:

1. Creamy Soup
2. Chicken a la Coconut
3. Beef Pho
4. Gazpacho
5. Cream of Spinach
6. Chilled Cucumber
7. Curried Cauliflower

Baked Goodies

Cassava Bread Loaf

Makes 1 loaf
Blood Type: all blood types
Step 1 (anti fungal)

What you will need: one 7½ x 3¾ x 2¼ inch loaf pan, 2 mixing bowls, 1 measuring cup, 1 set of measuring spoons

Ingredients

1½ cups cassava flour
½ tbsp tapioca flour
1¼ tbsp baking powder (without aluminium)
3 tbsp xylitol
1 tsp of salt
¼ cup heavy cream
2 eggs
⅓ cup olive oil
2oz butter

Method

- » Combine all dry ingredients except xylitol in large mixing bowl making sure that they are well mixed
- » Combine all wet ingredients including xylitol in small mixing bowl
- » Make a well in the dry ingredients and pour in the wet, folding the dry ingredients into the wet
- » Spoon dough into a greased and lined loaf pan

> Bake in oven at 350°F or 180°C for 30 minutes or until golden brown

This bread recipe is fabulous and simple and the versatility of choices of open-faced sandwiches that can be created is endless. Also add fresh herbs to the recipe for added flavour.

Cassava Crepes

Makes 6
Blood Type: all blood types
Step 1 (anti fungal)

What you will need: one 10 inch non-stick frying pan, one 6oz ladle, 2 mixing bowls, 1 measuring cup and 1 set of measuring spoons

Ingredients

2 cups cassava flour
1 tsp ground sea salt
2 eggs
1 cup olive oil
3 cups water

Method

- In large mixing bowl combine all of the dry ingredients
- In the medium bowl mix eggs, olive oil and 2 cups of water. Add to dry ingredients and mix well. Add more water if necessary to achieve a pouring consistency
- Heat non-stick frying pan and coat with a small amount of olive oil to prevent sticking
- Using 6oz ladle, pour mixture into pan moving the pan around to allow even coverage
- Allow to cook undisturbed until golden brown and then flip the crepe over to brown on the other side

These crepes are delicious topped with both savoury and sweet toppings. They may also be used as a wrap, just fill with meat and vegetable toppings. Dress with your favourite dressings and enjoy.

Pizza Crust Recipe

Makes 3 eight inch pizzas
Blood Type: all blood types
Step 1 (anti fungal)

What you will need: three 8 inch pizza pans, 1 measuring cup, 1 set of measuring spoons, 1 mixing bowl

Ingredients

3 cups cassava flour
2 eggs
⅔ tbsp baking powder (without aluminium)
⅓ cup olive oil
⅔ tbsp ground sea salt
½ cup water

Method

- » Combine all dry ingredients in large mixing bowl, making sure that they are well mixed
- » Make a well in the center and add wet ingredients. Fold the dry ingredients into the wet and knead until the dough is no longer sticking to the sides of the bowl, you may need to add a little more flour
- » Separate the dough into 3 and roll into balls on a floured surface dusting with flour as needed
- » Place one ball onto a lightly greased and floured pizza pans and press out to the sides
- » Bake at 350°F or 180°C for approximately 10 minutes or until golden brown
- » Repeat step 4 and 5 with the remaining balls of dough
- » Top with your favourite sauce and toppings and bake for a further 15 to 20 minutes or until cheese is melted

These pizza bases are so simple and you can create hundreds of varieties of breakfast, lunch and dinner ideas with this as a base.

Sauce

Ingredients

1 (6oz) can tomato paste natural and unsweetened
6 oz warm water
1 tsp minced garlic
2 tbsp agave nectar/xylitol
¼ tsp oregano
¾ tsp onion powder
¼ tsp marjoram
¼ tsp basil
¼ tsp ground black pepper
⅛ tsp red pepper flakes
Salt to taste

Method

In a small bowl, combine all ingredients. Mix well and allow to sit for 30 minutes to blend flavors, spread over pizza dough and prepare pizza as desired

Cassava Chocolate Cookies

Makes 18 Cookies
Blood Type: all blood types
Step 1 (anti fungal)

What you will need: 1 measuring cup, 2 cookie sheets, 1 electric mixer, 1 set of measuring spoons and 1 sieve

Ingredients

2 cups cassava flour
¼ cup tapioca flour
½ cup xylitol
12oz unsweetened cocoa powder
3 tbsp baking powder (without aluminum)
½ tsp salt
2 eggs
½ cup butter, softened
1 tsp organic vanilla/almond extract

Method

- » Preheat oven to 350°F or 180°C and line 2 cookie sheets with parchment paper
- » Whisk together all of dry ingredients except xylitol
- » In a large bowl, cream together butter and xylitol, until smooth, or for about 1 minute. (Use medium speed on a handheld or stand mixer.)
- » Add eggs, one at a time, mixing well between each addition. Add dry ingredients and extract; mix until dough forms
- » Drop rounded tablespoonfuls of dough onto the cookie sheets, about 2 inches apart
- » Bake first sheet for 10 to 12 minutes or until firm
- » Remove the sheet from oven and place on a wire rack to cool for 3 to 5 minutes then transfer cookies directly onto a rack to cool completely.
- » While first sheet is cooling, bake the second sheet of cookies. Once all cookies are cooled store them in an airtight container

Cheese Muffins

Makes 9 muffins
Blood Type: all blood types
Step 1 (anti fungal) Anabolic

What you will need: 1 muffin pan, 1 measuring cup, 1 set of measuring spoons, 1 electric mixer, 2 mixing bowls, 1 sieve

Ingredients

4 tbsp butter
1½ cups cassava flour
2 tsp baking powder
2 tsp xylitol
¼ tsp salt
1 tsp paprika
2 eggs
½ cup heavy cream
1 tsp dried thyme
2oz mozzarella cheese, cut into ½ inch cubes
2 tbsp Dijon mustard

Method

- » Preheat oven to 350°F or 180°C
- » Grease 9 muffin cups or use paper liners
- » Pour the mustard over cheese cubes and let sit for 5-10 mins
- » Melt butter and aside
- » In a mixing bowl, sift together flour, baking powder, xylitol, salt and paprika
- » In another bowl combine eggs, cream, melted butter and thyme and whisk to blend
- » Add the cream mixture to the other ingredients and stir just until moistened

- » Place heaped spoonful of batter into prepared cups, add a few pieces of cheese over each and top with another spoonful of batter
- » For even baking half fill any empty muffin cups with water
- » Bake until puffed and golden about 25 minutes. Allow to cool before removing from pan

Cassava Chocolate Cake

Makes 1 8-inch round cake or 24 cupcakes
Blood Type: all blood types
Step 1 (anti fungal)

What you will need: one 8 inch round pan, 1 measuring cup, 1 set of measuring spoons, 1 electric mixer, 1 mixing bowl

Ingredients

1½ cup cassava flour
½ cup tapioca flour
1 cup unsweetened cocoa powder
1½ tsp baking powder without aluminum
1½ tsp baking soda
1½ cups Xylitol
1 tsp salt
½ tsp xanthum gum
3 large eggs
½ cup cooking cream
½ cup water
½ cup olive oil
2 tsp organic vanilla extract
1 cup hot water

Method

» Preheat oven to 350°F or 180°C then grease and sprinkle the cocoa powder on 8 inch round pan or line 24 cupcake cups with paper liners
» In a large bowl, whisk together all dry ingredients
» Add eggs, cooking cream, ½ cup water, oil, and extract. Using an electric mixer beat for 2 minutes at medium speed. Turn the mixer to low, add hot water and mix for an additional minute
» Pour batter into prepared pan then bake. For 8-inch round pan, bake for 30 to 35 minutes. For cupcakes, bake for 18 to 20

minutes. A toothpick tester inserted into the center of any of the cakes should come out clean

- Remove pan(s) from the oven. Allow cake(s) to cool for 10 minutes in the pan and then turn them out onto a wire rack to cool completely
- Once cake is cool, ice as desired

Cassava Yellow Cake

Makes 1 8-inch round cake, or 18 cupcakes
Blood Type: all blood types
Step 1 (anti fungal)

What you will need: one 8 inch round pan, 1 measuring cup, 1 set of measuring spoons, 1 electric mixer, 2 mixing bowls

Ingredients

1½ cups cassava flour
⅓ cup tapioca flour
2 tsp baking powder (without aluminum)
½ tsp xanthum gum
1 tsp salt
4oz butter, softened
1 cup xylitol
4 large eggs
¾ cup cooking cream
2 tsp organic vanilla extract

Method

- » Preheat oven to 350°F or 180°C and grease 8-inch round pan, or line 18 cupcake pans with paper liners
- » In a medium bowl, whisk together all dry ingredients except xylitol
- » In another medium bowl, cream together butter and xylitol until light and fluffy, about 30 seconds. Use high speed on handheld mixer, medium-high on stand mixer.)
- » Add eggs and beat for an additional 15 seconds, the mixture will be very fluffy.
- » Add dry ingredients and mix until everything is well combined
- » Add cooking cream and vanilla extract. Blend until batter is thoroughly combined and fluffy
- » Pour batter into the prepared pans

- Bake until a toothpick tester inserted into the center of the cake comes out clean: For 8-inch round about 25 to 30; and for cupcakes about 20 to 25 minutes
- Remove the pan(s) from the oven and place them on wire racks to cool for 5 minutes. Transfer cake(s) directly onto the racks to cool completely
- Once cake is cool, ice as desired

Cassava Nachos

Makes 30
Blood Type: all blood types
Step 1 (anti fungal)

What you will need: one 10 inch non-stick frying pan, one 6oz ladle, 2 mixing bowls, 1 measuring cup, 1 pizza cutter and 1 set of measuring spoons

Ingredients

2 cups cassava flour
1 tsp ground sea salt
2 eggs
1 cup olive oil
3 cups water
1 tbsp Italian seasoning
1 tbsp basil
1 tbsp parsley
1 tsp black pepper

Method

- In large mixing bowl combine all of the dry ingredients
- In medium bowl mix eggs, olive oil and 2 cups of water. Add to dry ingredients and mix well. Add more water if necessary to achieve a pouring consistency
- Heat non-stick frying pan and coat with a small amount of olive oil to prevent sticking
- Using 6oz ladle, pour mixture into pan moving the pan around to allow even coverage
- Allow to cook undisturbed until golden brown and then flip the crepe over to brown on the other side
- Remove from pan, allow to cool and slice into eight equal parts
- Deep fry each section until golden brown and crispy
- Serve with one of the delicious dips from the dips section

Dressings

Although not entirely a wheat-based food item, we have found that many salad dressings have other unnatural ingredients in them. Salad dressings are meant to be as delicious and natural as the salad itself. We have included in this section directions for making an excellent salad dressing that contains antifungal ingredients. Eating a regular salad daily while on the program is an excellent way of improving the mineral and vitamin levels of the body through living plants.

Antifungal Salad Dressing/ Gentle Liver Flush

Serves 4
Blood Type: all blood types
Step 1 (anti fungal) Catabolic

Ingredients

1 cup olive oil
3 cloves garlic, chopped
Pinch of dried ginger
Juice of 1 lemon
3 tsp apple cider vinegar
Pinch sea salt
A few leaves fresh basil and chives, to taste
1 tbsp xylitol

Method

- » Blend all the ingredients together and drizzle on salads and vegetables as a delicious accompanying sauce or dressing

The above dressing can also be used as a mild liver/gall bladder flush. You should consume four to six ounces of neat unsweetened apple juice for one week prior to the flush to clean the liver and gall bladder. Apple juice, with its high malic acid content, inhibits fungal growth, and it helps to dissolve gallstones. The dressing should be taken neat if it is used as a liver/gall bladder flush. The dose is one-third cup per day for ten days. Keep the meals light and healthy.

Fresh Lemon & Coriander Dressing

Serves 4
Blood Type: all blood types
Step 1 (anti fungal) Catabolic

Ingredients

1 tbsp fresh lemon juice
1-2 cloves garlic, crushed
½ tsp each of ground cumin & ground coriander
Sea salt & freshly ground black pepper
6 tbsp light olive oil

Method

- » Place the lemon juice, garlic, ground spices, and salt and pepper to taste, in a small bowl and whisk together until thoroughly mixed. Gradually whisk in the oil until well mixed and thickened. Whisk in a little extra lemon juice, if desired
- » Alternatively, place all the ingredients in a clean screw top jar, seal and shake well until thoroughly mixed
- » Adjust the seasoning to taste and serve immediately, or keep in a screw top jar in the refrigerator for up to 3 days. Whisk or shake thoroughly before serving

Sweet Basil Dressing

Serves 6
Blood Type: all blood types
Step 1 (anti fungal) Catabolic

Ingredients

6 tbsp unsweetened white grape juice
4 tbsp olive oil
2 tbsp cider vinegar
2-3 tbsp chopped fresh basil
1 clove garlic, crushed
A pinch of xylitol
Sea salt & freshly ground black pepper

Method

- Place the grape juice, olive oil, vinegar, chopped basil, garlic, xylitol and seasoning in a small bowl and whisk together until thoroughly mixed
- Alternatively, place all the ingredients in a clean screw-top jar in the refrigerator for up to 3 days. Whisk or shake thoroughly before serving
- Adjust the seasoning to taste and serve immediately, or keep in a screw-top jar in the refrigerator for up to 3 days. Whisk or shake thoroughly before serving

Mixed Herb Yoghurt Dressing

Serves 4
Blood Type: all blood types
Step 1 (anti fungal) Anabolic

Ingredients

50 oz (¼ pint) natural yogurt or natural Greek yogurt
2 tsp fresh lemon juice
A pinch of xylitol
2 small cloves garlic, crushed
2 tbsp chopped fresh mixed herbs, such as parsley, oregano, thyme & chives
Sea salt & freshly ground black pepper

Method

- » Place all the ingredients in a small bowl and mix together until well blended
- » Adjust the seasoning to taste, then serve immediately, or cover and chill for 1-2 hours before serving

Herby Mustard Dressing

Serves 4
Blood Type: all blood types
Step 1 (anti fungal) Catabolic

Ingredients

3 tbsp olive oil
3 tbsp cider vinegar
1 tbsp wholegrain mustard (unsweetened & natural)
1 clove garlic, crushed
1 tbsp chopped fresh parsley
1 tbsp snipped fresh chives
Sea salt & freshly ground black pepper

Method

- » Put the oil, vinegar, mustard, garlic and chopped herbs in a small bowl and whisk together until thoroughly mixed. Season to taste with salt and pepper
- » Alternatively, put all the ingredients in a clean screw-top jar, seal and shake well until thoroughly mixed
- » Adjust the seasoning and serve immediately, or keep in a screw-top jar in the refrigerator for up to 3 days. Whisk or shake thoroughly before serving

Creamy Curried Dressing

Serves 6
Blood Type: all blood types
Step 1 (anti fungal) Anabolic

Ingredients

6 tbsp homemade mayonnaise (see recipe in DIPS section)
4 tbsp natural yogurt
2 tbsp natural Greek yogurt
1 tbsp tomato purée (unsweetened & natural)
1 tbsp medium-hot curry paste
2 tbsp snipped fresh chives
Sea salt & freshly ground black pepper

Method

- » Place the mayonnaise, yogurts, tomato purée, curry paste and snipped chives in a small bowl and stir together until well mixed
- » Season to taste with salt and pepper. Serve cold. Store in a covered container in the refrigerator for up to 2 days

Salsas & Pestos

Salsa Verde

Serves 4
Blood Type: all blood types
Step 1 (anti fungal) Catabolic

Ingredients

½ cup finely chopped fresh flat-leaf parsley
¼ cup finely chopped fresh dill
¼ cup finely chopped fresh chives
1 tbsp wholegrain mustard
2 tbsp lemon juice
2 tbsp drained, rinsed baby capers, chopped finely
1 clove garlic, crushed
1/3 cup olive oil
Sea salt & freshly ground black pepper (to spice it up use red chili flakes)

Method

- » Combine ingredients in a small bowl (chill before serving). Add sea salt & freshly ground black pepper to taste

Salsa Verde goes great with steaks, grilled lamb cutlets; poached salmon fillets. Or roasted chicken breasts. Vary your proteins flavor every night by changing your dressing, sauce or pesto.

Mango & Avocado Salsa

Serves 4
Blood Type: all blood types
Step 2 Anabolic

Ingredients

1 medium mango (roughly chopped)
1 large avocado (roughly chopped)
1 small red onion (roughly chopped)
1 small red pepper (finely chopped)
2 tablespoon of lime juice
1 fresh thai chili
Sea salt & freshly ground black pepper (to taste)

Method

> » Combine all of the ingredients in a bowl (chill before serving). Add sea salt & freshly ground black pepper to taste

Mango salsa goes on its own with cassava crackers, cassava chips, sweet potato chips (Step 2) & is also delicious on top of grilled or blackened fish. Vary your proteins flavor every night by changing your dressing, sauce or pesto.

Classic Basil Pesto

Serves 4
Blood Type: all blood types
Step 1 (anti fungal) Catabolic

Ingredients

2 cups firmly packed fresh basil leaves
2 cloves garlic, quartered
1/3 cup roasted pine nuts
½ cup crumbled feta cheese
¾ cup olive oil
Sea salt & freshly ground black pepper (to spice it up use red chili flakes)

Method

» Blend or process basil, garlic, nuts and cheese until chopped finely. With motor operating, gradually add oil in thin, steady stream; process until smooth. Add sea salt & freshly ground black pepper to taste

Basil Pesto is so versatile. Use as a spread, use on your pizza bases, top your gluten free pasta, lamb, beef & fish. . Vary your proteins flavor every night by changing your dressing, sauce or pesto.

Rocket & Mint with Macadamia

Serves 4
Blood Type: all blood types
Step 1 (anti fungal) Catabolic

Ingredients

½ cup firmly packed fresh mint leaves
1.4 oz baby rocket leaves
½ cup roasted macadamias
¼ cup crumbled feta cheese
2 cloves garlic, quartered
1 tablespoon lemon juice
2 tablespoons water
½ cup olive oil
Sea salt & freshly ground black pepper (to spice it up use red chili flakes)

Method

» Blend or process mint, rocket, nuts, cheese, garlic, juice and water until combined. With motor operating, gradually add oil in thin, steady stream; process until smooth. Add sea salt & freshly ground black pepper to taste

This pesto version is great with gluten free pasta, sweet potato salad & as a marinade for all kebabs. Vary your proteins flavor every night by changing your dressing, sauce or pesto.

Red Pepper Pesto

Serves 4
Blood Type: all blood types
Step 1 (anti fungal) Anabolic (p.m)/Catabolic (a.m)

Ingredients

1 large red capsicum (12 oz), roasted, peeled
½ cup drained semi-dried tomatoes
½ cup firmly packed fresh basil leaves
2 tablespoons roasted pine nuts
¼ cup crumbled feta cheese
½ cup olive oil
Sea salt & freshly ground black pepper (to spice it up use red chili flakes)

Method

» Blend or process capsicum, tomatoes, basil, nuts, and cheese until chopped. With motor operating, gradually add oil in thin, steady stream; process until smooth. Add sea salt & freshly ground black pepper to taste

Red pepper pesto is great on chicken & fish and also as a marinade. Vary your proteins flavor every night by changing your dressing, sauce or pesto.

Dips

Homemade Mayonnaise

Makes 20 oz
Blood Type: all blood types
Step 1 (anti fungal) Anabolic

Ingredients

2 egg yolks
1 egg (whole)
1 tbsp French style mustard (unsweetened & natural)
Pinch of white or red pepper
Pinch of salt
Juice of lemon (or part of)
2 cups of olive oil

Method

- Put the first 6 ingredients in a bowl or in your processor
- Drizzle in your oil until desired consistency is achieved, whisking or blending continuously
- Taste your mayonnaise. You might want to add a bit more lemon juice or salt. Also remember that real mayonnaise is art so be artistic and add other seasonings such as curry or tarragon, chili, dill or any other herb or spice

Guacamole

Serves 4-6
Blood Type: all blood types
Step 1 (anti fungal) Catabolic

Ingredients

2 ripe avocados
Juice of 1 small lime
3 shallots, finely chopped
2 plum tomatoes, skinned, seeded & finely chopped
1 fresh green chili, seeded & finely chopped
1 clove garlic, crushed
1 tbsp chopped fresh coriander
Sea salt & freshly ground black pepper
Fresh coriander sprigs, to garnish

Method

- » Halve, stone and peel the avocados and place the flesh in a bowl. Mash the avocado flesh with the limejuice until smooth
- » Stir in the shallots, tomatoes, chili, garlic, chopped coriander and salt and pepper to taste. Mix well
- » Transfer the mixture to a bowl, garnish with coriander sprigs and serve immediately

Guacamole goes well with cassava crackers, cassava chips, sweet potato chips (Step 2) & other gluten free breads.

Coriander Hummus

Serves 4
Blood Type: all blood types
Step 1 (anti fungal) Anabolic (p.m)/Catabolic (a.m)

Ingredients

15oz can chick peas, rinsed & drained
Juice of lemon
3 tbsp extra-virgin olive oil
2 tbsp light tahini paste
1 clove garlic, crushed
½ tsp ground coriander
½ tsp ground cumin
Sea salt & freshly ground black pepper
Fresh coriander sprigs, to garnish

Method

- » Place the chick-peas in a blender or food processor with the lemon juice, olive oil, tahini paste, garlic, ground cumin, and salt and pepper to taste. Blend until smooth and thoroughly mixed. Adjust the seasoning to taste
- » Transfer the mixture to a bowl. Garnish with coriander sprigs and serve

Coriander Hummus goes great with cassava crackers, cassava chips, sweet potato chips (Step 2) & other gluten free breads or vegetable crudités.

Tzatziki

Serves 4
Blood Type: all blood types
Step 1 (anti fungal) Anabolic (p.m)/Catabolic (a.m)

Ingredients

1 large cucumber
10 oz (½ pint) natural Greek yogurt
1 tbsp light olive oil
2 cloves garlic, crushed
2 tbsp chopped fresh mint
a squeeze of fresh lemon
a pinch of xylitol
Sea salt & freshly ground black pepper

Method

- » Halve, deseed and finely chop the cucumber. Place the cucumber in a bowl, add the yogurt and olive oil and stir to mix well
- » Add the garlic and chopped mint, lemon and xylitol and mix well, then season to taste with salt and pepper. Cover and chill until ready to serve

Tzatziki is fabulous with cassava crackers, cassava chip, sweet potato chips (Step 2) & other gluten free breads & can also be served as a side dish for spicy Eastern flavoured dishes.

Watercress Cheese Dip

Serves 6
Blood Type: all blood types
Step 1 (anti fungal) Anabolic

Ingredients

8oz full-fat soft cheese
3 tbsp crème fraîche
2.5 oz watercress, finely chopped
1 clove garlic, crushed
a squeeze of fresh lemon
Sea salt & freshly ground black pepper (to spice it up use red chili flakes)

Method

- » Place the soft cheese in a bowl and stir until softened a little more. Stir in the crème fraîche until well combined
- » Stir in the watercress, lemon and garlic, then season to taste with salt and pepper
- » Cover and chill for at least 1 hour before serving, to allow the flavors to develop

Watercress cheese dip goes great with raw vegetable crudités as well as cassava crackers, cassava chips or sweet potato chips (Step 2) & other gluten free bread.

Sour Cream & Chive Dip

Serves 6
Blood Type: all blood types
Step 1 (anti fungal) Anabolic

Ingredients

10 oz (½ pint) thick soured cream or crème fraîche
1 clove garlic, crushed
2-3 spring onions, finely chopped
3-4 tbsp snipped fresh chives
Sea salt & freshly ground black pepper (to spice it up use red chili flakes)
Fresh chive flowers, to garnish (optional)

Method

- » Place the soured cream or crème fraîche in a bowl. Add the garlic, spring onions, lemon and snipped chives and mix well. Season to taste with salt and pepper
- » Transfer the mixture to a bowl and serve immediately, or cover and chill until ready to serve. Garnish with chive flowers just before serving, if desired

Sour cream and chive dip is so diverse in its uses. Serve with raw vegetable crudités or on top of roasted ground provisions as well as being great with cassava crackers, cassava chips, sweet potato chips (Step 2) & other gluten free bread.

Quick Snacks

Chocolate & Fruit Crackles

Makes 24
Blood Type: all blood types
Step 2 Anabolic

Ingredients

2 cups gluten-free cornflakes
1 cup puffed rice
½ cup raisins
⅓ cup almond meal
2 tbsp sunflower seeds
8.8oz unsweetened chocolate, melted
2 tablespoons of xylitol

Method

- » Line your two 12-hole flat-based patty pans with paper cases
- » Combine your cornflakes, rice, raisins, almond meal and seeds in a large bowl and stir in your melted chocolate that has been combined with the xylitol
- » Spoon your mixture among the paper cases and press down gently. For a finished look sprinkle the tray with powdered xylitol sugar. You can make fine xylitol to form an 'icing sugar' presentation by placing it in your food processor or blender. Refrigerate for 1 hour or until they have set

Dried fruit and coconut trail mix

Makes 3 cups
Blood Type: all blood types
Step 2 Anabolic

Ingredients

2 tbsp agave syrup
2 tsp olive oil
¼ tsp mixed spice
½ cup finely chopped pecans
½ cup almond kernels
½ cup toasted flaked coconut
½ cup craisins
½ cup coarsely chopped dried apricots
½ cup coarsely chopped dried dates

Method

- » Preheat oven to 350°F/180°C
- » Combine your agave syrup, oil and spices into a small bowl
- » Combine your nuts into a shallow baking dish and drizzle with the agave mixture. Roast the tray uncovered for about 10 minutes or until browned lightly, giving it a gentle stir halfway through cooking time. Allow to cool for at least 15 minutes
- » Stir in the remaining ingredients and then fully cool

Mozzarella Crisps

Makes 18
Blood Type: all blood types
Step 1 Anabolic

Ingredients

1 cup finely grated mozzarella cheese
¼ tsp finely ground black pepper
1 tsp dried oregano

Method

- » Preheat your oven to 350°F/180°C
- » Combine all of your ingredients into a medium bowl. Place 2 tsp of the mixture, 3cm apart, onto baking-paper-lined oven trays and flatten each patty with your fingertips
- » Bake them uncovered for about 4 minutes and cool on trays. Keep an eye on them as they crisp fast

Oven-baked Vegetable Crisps

Serves 8
Blood Type: all blood types
Step 1 Anabolic

Ingredients

Coconut -oil spray
1 kg parsnips
28oz cassava
14oz sweet potato (step 2 only)
2 tsp sea salt
Paprika to sprinkle
Fresh finely chopped parsley

Method

- Preheat oven to 320°F/160°C fan-forced and spray three oven trays with the coconut oil spray
- Using mandolin, v-slicer or sharp knife, cut the parsnip, cassavas and sweet potatoes into 2mm slices
- Place the parsnips, in a single layer, on oven trays and lightly coat with the coconut oil spray., salt and paprika and then bake, uncovered for about 40 minutes or until browned on both sides and crisp. Turn them onto a wire rack to cool
- Repeat the process another 2 times using the cassavas then the sweet potatoes
- Sprinkle crisps with the finely chopped parsley

Mini Pizzava Squares

Makes 40 squares
Blood Type: all blood types
Step 1 Anabolic

Ingredients

See Pizza Crust recipe in The Baked Goods Section for the crust
⅓ cup tomato paste (natural and unsweetened)
2 medium tomatoes, thinly sliced
9.5oz grilled capsicum, chopped coarsely
½ small red onion, sliced thinly
5.2oz soft feta cheese, crumbled
15.5oz pineapple chunks **(Step 2 only)**
3.5oz turkey, chopped coarsely
1 cup mozzarella cheese
½ cup seeded green olives, halved
20 small fresh basil leaves
5 cherry tomatoes, quartered
20 fresh oregano leaves

Method

- Preheat oven to 390°F/200°C fan-forced and oil two 25cm x 35cm pans
- Line bases with baking paper, extending paper 5cm over long sides
- Mix your pizza crusts according to the recipe in the Baked Goods Section and spread your mixture into the pans
- Bake them for about 12 minutes or until browned lightly and then remove from the oven
- Spread homemade paste over crusts and sprinkle sliced tomato, capsicum, onion, and feta over one pizzava base
- Sprinkle pineapple (Step 2 only), turkey and mozzarella cheese over your remaining pizzava crust

- » Bake your pizzavas for about 15 minutes or until the cheese melts and bases are crisp. Cut each pizzava into 20 squares.
- » Top each capsicum and feta pizzava square with olives and basil leaves. Top each turkey and pineapple pizzava square with a cherry tomato chunk and oregano leaves

Herbed Mahi-Mahi Kebabs

Serves 8
Blood Type: all blood types
Step 1 Catabolic

Ingredients

2 kg mahi-mahi steaks (70oz)
4 medium lemons (19oz)
⅓ cup finely chopped fresh coriander
½ cup finely chopped fresh flat-leaf parsley
½ cup finely chopped fresh chives
½ tsp freshly ground black pepper
2 tbsp coconut oil

Method

- Remove and discard the skin from the fish and cut into 3cm pieces
- Using your zester, remove as much of the rind as possible from the lemons and squeeze ⅔ cup juice from the lemons
- Combine your fish rind, juice, herbs, pepper and oil in large bowl
- Weave your fish onto 16 skewers and then place them in single layer, in large shallow dish. Pour any of your remaining marinade over the skewers and then cover and refrigerate for at least 3 hours or overnight
- Cook the marinated skewers on a heated and oiled grill plate (or grill or barbecue) until browned all over and cooked through
- Serve with baby spinach leaves, a mesclun salad and a delicious dip like Tzatziki found in the Dips Section

Beef and Onion Kebabs

Serves 4
Blood Type: O, B
Step 1 Anabolic served warm/Catabolic served cold

Ingredients

700g beef rump steak
18 baby onions (450g), halved
Marinade
½ cup tomato sauce natural and unsweetened
½ cup agave syrup **(replace with Xylitol on Step 1)**
½ cup lemon juice, rind also optional for added flavour
2 tbsp finely chopped fresh oregano
4cm piece fresh ginger (20g), grated
1 tbsp tamari sauce

Method

- » Make marinade
- » Cut beef into 3cm pieces
- » Thread beef and onion, alternately, onto 12 skewers. Place kebabs in a shallow dish, add marinade and refrigerate for a minimum of 3 hours or overnight
- » Cook kebabs on heated and oiled grill plate (or grill or barbecue), uncovered, until browned and cooked as desired
- » These can be served with a mesclun salad and the delicious Rocket and Mint with Macadamia Pesto in the Dips Section
- » **Marinade** Combine ingredients in medium jug

Chicken Tikka Masala Drumsticks

Serves 4
Blood Type: O, A
Step 1 Anabolic served warm/Catabolic served cold

Ingredients

12 chicken drumettes
⅓ cup tikka masala paste
½ cup yogurt
¼ cup coarsely chopped fresh coriander
2 pinches of xylitol
small amount of grated lemon zest

Method

- » Preheat your oven to moderately hot
- » Place chicken in large bowl with combined paste and 2 tbsp of the yogurt and the pinches of xylitol then toss to coat the chicken into a paste mixture
- » Place the chicken in a single layer, on a wire rack in large baking dish. Roast, uncovered, in a moderately hot oven for about 20 minutes or until chicken is browned and cooked through
- » Meanwhile, combine the coriander and remaining yogurt in small bowl with a pinch of xylitol and small amount of grated lemon zest
- » Serve your chicken drizzled with the divine yogurt mixture, and accompanied by oven baked vegetable chips and lime pickle

Breakfast Ideas

Eggs Florentine

Serves 1
Blood Type: all blood types
Step 1 Anabolic (p.m)/Catabolic(a.m)

Ingredients

3½ -7oz fresh spinach
1 tbsp water
1 tsp apple cider vinegar
1 large or 2 small eggs
Freshly grated nutmeg
Salt and pepper

Method

- » Wash the spinach and place in a large saucepan with the water. Cover and cook over a medium heat for 1-2 minutes, until wilted. Season to taste
- » When it has become soft, cut through the spinach roughly with a sharp knife then and transfer it to a warmed serving plate
- » Meanwhile, set a frying pan on the stove and pour in boiling water to a depth of about 2.5cm (1 inch). Keep the water at a gentle rolling boil
- » Add the vinegar to hold eggs together. Crack each egg into a saucer and slip it gently into the boiling water. Cook just long enough to set the white while the yolk remains runny
- » Remove the poached egg with a slotted spoon and slide onto spinach
- » Season with plenty of nutmeg, salt and pepper

Belgian Waffles

Makes 5 to 7 Waffles
Blood Type: all blood types
Step 1 Anabolic

Ingredients

¾ cup cassava flour
¼ cup tapioca flour
1 tsp baking powder (without aluminum)
½ tsp salt
½ tsp baking soda
1 tsp xylitol
3 large eggs
1 cup cooking cream
4 tbsp butter, melted

Method

- » In a medium bowl, whisk together all dry ingredients
- » In a small bowl, whisk together wet ingredients and pour over dry ingredients
- » Blend until everything is thoroughly combined
- » Bake in waffle iron according to appliance instructions
- » Serve immediately with powdered xylitol
- » Add fresh organic berries for added flavour

NB: can be made in both standard and Belgian waffle iron.

Warm Bean Salad

Serves 1-2
Blood Type: all blood types
Step 2 Anabolic (p.m)/Catabolic (a.m)

Ingredients

4 oz okra, thickly sliced
1 large garlic clove, crushed
5-6 tbsp water
3-4 tbsp canned butter beans, drained and rinsed
3-4 tbsp canned red kidney beans, drained and rinsed
1 tsp lemon or lime juice
1 tsp olive oil
1 small handful of fresh parsley, coriander, dill, tarragon and pepper
1 thick slice of crusty cassava bread, to serve

Method

- » Place the okra, garlic and water in a small saucepan. Cover and heat until boiling, then simmer gently for 3-4 minutes until soft, drain
- » Meanwhile, heat the butter beans and red kidney beans with the lemon or lime juice over a gentle heat, strain
- » Add the okra and garlic with the olive oil, herbs and a little black pepper
- » Stir gently and serve with a thick slice of crusty cassava bread, which you can use to mop up the delicious juices

Green Bean & Egg Salad

Serves 2
Blood Type: all blood types
Step 1 Anabolic (p.m)/Catabolic (a.m)

Ingredients

8oz green beans, roughly chopped
6-8 cherry tomatoes, halved
2 garlic cloves, finely chopped
2 tsp toasted almond nuts
2 tsp olive oil
4 tsp apple cider vinegar
2 eggs, hard boiled and chopped
Black pepper
2 slices of cassava bread, to serve

Method

- » Cook the beans (or other vegetables) briskly in a saucepan of boiling water for 5-10 minutes, until tender
- » Drain vegetables well and return them to the saucepan
- » Add the halved cherry tomatoes, garlic, a little black pepper, almond nuts, olive oil and Apple Cider vinegar
- » Stir gently to combine, add the chopped hard-boiled egg and stir gently again
- » Serve warm with cassava bread

Tomato & Courgette Bake

Serves 2
Blood Type: all blood types
Step 1 Anabolic

Ingredients

7 oz small vine tomatoes, halved
2 small courgettes
2 tsp olive oil
2 tsp chopped thyme
2 garlic cloves, finely chopped
4 eggs
3 tbsp cooking cream
2 tbsp freshly grated mozzarella cheese
Salt and pepper
Salad leaves, to serve

Method

- » Lightly oil a 900 ml shallow ovenproof dish or two individual dishes
- » Scatter with the tomatoes, courgettes, thyme and garlic and season lightly with salt and pepper
- » Add oil and toss to mix everything together well
- » Bake in preheated oven, 200°C, for 10 minutes
- » Lightly beat eggs with cooking cream and salt and pepper to taste, pour mixture over the vegetables
- » Sprinkle with cheese and bake for a further 30 minutes until golden and lightly set. Serve with organic salad greens.

Omelet Wrap with Stir Fried Greens

Serves 4
Blood Type:
Step 1 Anabolic

Ingredients

5oz broccoli cut into small florets
2 tbsp coconut/olive oil
1½cm piece of fresh root ginger, finely grated
1 large garlic clove, crushed
2 fresh red chillies, seeded and finely sliced
4 spring onions (scallions), sliced diagonally
6oz shredded pak choi (bok choy)
2oz fresh coriander (cilantro) leaves, plus extra to garnish
4oz bean sprouts
3 tbsp tamari soy sauce
4 eggs
Sea Salt and ground pepper

Method

- Blanch the broccoli in salted boiling water for
- 2 minutes. Drain and refresh under cold water, then drain again
- In the meantime, heat 1 tbsp of oil in a large frying pan or wok. Stir-fry the ginger, garlic and half the chilli for 1 minute
- Add spring onions, broccoli and pak choi. Toss the ingredients over the heat for 2 minutes
- Chop three-quarters of the coriander and add to pan or wok, with bean sprouts. Stir-fry for 1 minute, then add tamari soy sauce and heat through for 1 minute more
- Remove pan from the heat and it keep warm
- Beat eggs lightly with a fork and season well. Heat a little of the remaining oil in a small frying pan and add one-quarter of the beaten egg
- Swirl the pan so the egg spreads to cover the base, then sprinkle over one-quarter of the reserved coriander leaves

- » Cook until just set, then turn the omelet out onto a plate and keep warm while you make three more omelets, adding more oil when necessary
- » Spoon the vegetable stir-fry onto the omelets and gently roll them up. Cut them in half crossways and serve on individual plates, garnished with the extra coriander leaves and the remaining chili

Light Lunch Salads

Salmon and Avocado Salad

Serves 4
Blood Type: all blood types
Step 1 Anabolic (p.m)/Catabolic (a.m)

Ingredients

7oz frozen broad beans
7oz baby spinach leaves
7oz trimmed celery stalks, sliced thinly
2 medium avocados, peeled, sliced
1½ cups water
1½ cups fish stock
¼ cup apple cider vinegar
4 dill stalks
6 whole black peppercorns
1 clove garlic, halved
8oz skinless salmon fillets

Dill and Mustard Dressing
1 clove garlic, crushed
½ cup olive oil
¼ cup apple cider vinegar
2 tsp Dijon mustard (natural and unsweetened)
1 tsp finely chopped fresh dill

Method

- » Boil or steam beans until just tender and drain, removing and discarding the outer shells
- » Combine beans, spinach, celery and avocado in large bowl
- » Make simple dill and mustard dressing

- » Combine water, stock, dill, peppercorns and garlic in a large shallow frying pan and bring to a gentle simmer
- » Add salmon to the pan and simmer gently, uncovered for around 5 minutes or until cooked as desired, remembering to turn the salmon over halfway through cooking
- » Drain salmon from the pan, and transfer to a plate. Using two forks, flake cooked salmon into large pieces. Gently toss salmon with the delicious bean mixture and half of the dill and mustard dressing
- » Serve green salad drizzled with the remaining dressing

Dill and mustard dressing place ingredients in screw-top jar and shake well

Mediterranean Chicken Salad

Serves 4
Blood Type: O, A
Step 1 Anabolic served warm/Catabolic served cold

Ingredients

2 cups chicken stock
4 single chicken breasts fillets (23oz)
2 medium yellow capsicums (14oz)
1 large loaf cassava bread (17½oz)
3½oz butter, melted
2 cloves garlic, crushed
1 tbsp finely chopped fresh flat-leaf parsley
7oz baby rocket leaves
8½oz teardrop tomatoes, halved
⅓ cup black olives

Anchovy dressing

½ cup firmly packed fresh basil leaves
½ cup extra virgin olive oil
2 tbsp finely feta cheese
2 drained anchovy fillets
1 tbsp lemon juice

Method

- » Preheat your oven to a very high heat
- » Pour your stock into a medium frying pan and bring it to a boil. Add chicken and simmer, loosely covered for about 8 minutes, turning halfway, until chicken is properly cooked through
- » Remove chicken from pan and allow to stand for 10 minutes before slicing
- » In the meantime, quarter your capsicums, removing and discarding the seeds and membranes

- » Roast them in very hot oven or under a hot grill, skin side up, until the skin blisters and blackens
- » Cover the capsicum pieces with plastic or paper for 5 minutes; then peel away the skin and slice the capsicum
- » Reduce the oven temperature to moderately hot
- » Remove most of the crust from the cassava bread, cut them into 1.5cm slices then cut them into 3cm pieces.
- » Divide bread pieces between two oven trays. Drizzle over the combined melted butter, garlic and parsley and toss gently to coat all bread pieces
- » Bake the cassava bread pieces in a moderately hot oven for about 10 minutes or until browned lightly
- » In the meantime make your scrumptious anchovy dressing
- » Arrange your rocket, tomato, olives, chicken and capsicum on a serving platter and just before serving, toss through your croutons and drizzle lavishly with anchovy dressing

Anchovy dressing Blend your ingredients until the dressing is completely smooth.

Sesame Chicken Salad

Serves 4
Blood Type: O, A
Step 1 Anabolic served warm/Catabolic served cold

Ingredients

5oz snow peas
4 cups shredded and flavoured/spiced pre-cooked chicken
3½oz snow pea sprouts
2 cups bean sprouts
2 trimmed sticks celery, sliced thinly
4 green onions, sliced thinly
1 tbsp roasted sesame seeds
Sea salt and course ground black pepper to taste (choose red chili flakes for extra zing)

Dressing

2 tbsp coconut oil
2 tsp sesame oil
½ tsp five-spice powder
2 tbsp tamari soy
1 tbsp lime-juice
Sea salt and course ground black pepper to taste (choose red chili flakes for extra zing)

Method

- » Place your snow peas in a medium sized bowl. Cover with boiling water and drain immediately
- » Cover snow peas with cold water in the same bowl and allow to stand for 2 minutes. Drain and thinly slice
- » Combine snow peas in large bowl with chicken, snow pea sprouts, bean sprouts, celery, onion and dressing. Toss them all gently to combine all of the ingredients thoroughly
- » Sprinkle this divine salad with sesame seeds to serve
- » Dressing Combine ingredients in screw-top jar and shake it well

Nicoise Salad

Serves 4
Blood Type: all blood types
Step 1/ 2 Anabolic (p.m)/Catabolic (a.m)

Ingredients

7oz baby green beans, trimmed
3 medium tomatoes, cut into wedges
4 hard-boiled eggs, quartered
15oz can tuna in spring-water, drained, rinsed
½ cup drained caper-berries, rinsed
½ cup seeded small black olives
¼ cup firmly packed fresh flat-leaf parsley
15oz cassava/yam, diced
2 tbsp olive oil
1 tbsp lemon juice
2 tbsp apple cider vinegar
Sea salt and course ground black pepper to taste (choose red chili flakes for extra zing)

Method

- » Boil or steam your beans until they become just tender then immediately drain them. Rinse them thoroughly under cold water and drain again.
- » Meanwhile, combine your tomatoes, eggs, flaked tuna, caper berries, olives, parsley and cassava/yam in large bowl.
- » Combine all of your remaining ingredients in screw-top jar and then shake well. Add your beans to this fabulous salad, drizzle with dressing and toss gently to combine.

Roast beef and rocket salad

Serves 4
Blood Type: O, B
Step 1 Anabolic served warm/Catabolic served cold

Ingredients

1 tbsp olive oil
21oz piece beef eye fillet
2 tbsp fresh tarragon
17½oz cassava/yam
4oz semi-dried tomatoes
3½ baby rocket leaves
3½oz red onion, sliced thinly
½ cup cooking cream
⅓ cup homemade mayonnaise
1 tbsp Dijon mustard (natural and unsweetened)
2 cloves garlic, crushed
Sea salt and course ground black pepper to taste (choose red chili flakes for extra zing)

Method

- » Preheat your oven to moderate heat
- » Heat oil in a medium flameproof baking dish and cook beef with tarragon, garlic and salt and pepper to taste, frequently turning, until browned nicely
- » Roast, uncovered, in moderately hot oven for about 15 minutes or until it is cooked as desired
- » Remove meat from oven, cover and leave to stand for at least 5 minutes, then slice beef thinly
- » Meanwhile, boil or steam your cassava/yam or both (diced into small cubes) until well tender and drain thoroughly
- » Combine thinly sliced beef and cassava/yam in a large bowl with tomato, rocket and onions
- » Combine all remaining ingredients in screw-top jar and shake well. Drizzle the dressing liberally over salad and toss gently to combine

Vegetable, Haloumi and Rocket Salad

Serves 4
Blood Type: all blood types
Step 1 Catabolic

Ingredients

8½oz haloumi cheese, cut into 2cm cubes
1 medium red capsicum, chopped coarsely
1 medium yellow capsicum, chopped coarsely
2 medium zucchini, sliced thickly
6oz fresh asparagus
2 tbsp fresh oregano
a sprinkle of paprika
2 tbsp olive oil
2 tbsp apple cider vinegar
1 clove garlic, crushed
5oz baby rocket leaves
Fresh mixed herbs
Sea salt and course ground black pepper to taste (choose red chili flakes for extra zing)

Method

- » Cook cheese, capsicums, asparagus and zucchini, in batches on a heated oiled grill plate (or grill or barbecue) until browned lightly and just tender
- » Sprinkle fresh oregano and paprika to flavour the cheese and vegetables lightly, repeat process while cooking
- » Meanwhile, place your oil, vinegar, fresh mixed herbs and garlic in a screw top jar and shake well
- » Combine cheese and vegetables in large bowl with rocket and dressing then toss all of ingredients gently to fully combine the flavours before serving

Fish Burritos

Serves 8
Blood Type: all blood types
Step 1 Anabolic (p.m)/Catabolic (a.m)

Ingredients

1 cup coarsely chopped fresh coriander
2 tsp finely chopped coriander root and stem mixture
1 fresh long red chilli, chopped coarsely
1 clove garlic, quartered
1½ tsp sweet paprika
1 tsp ground cumin
⅓ cup olive oil
28oz small white fish fillets, halved
8x20cm round cassava crepes **(see recipe in Baked Goodies Section)**
1 baby cos lettuce (6oz), leaves separated
1 Lebanese cucumber (4½oz), sliced thinly
Sea salt and course ground black pepper to taste (choose red chili flakes for extra zing)

Lime buttermilk dressing

¼ cup buttermilk
1 tsp finely grated lime rind
2 tsp lime juice
Sea salt and course ground black pepper to taste (choose red chili flakes for extra zing)

Method

- » Blend or food process coriander leaves, root and stem mixture, chili, garlic, paprika, cumin and ¼ cup of oil until it is all smooth
- » Combine your coriander mixture and fish in large bowl, cover and refrigerate for a minimum of 30 minutes
- » Meanwhile, make delicious lime buttermilk dressing
- » Heat remaining oil in a large frying pan and cook pre-marinated fish in batches, until lightly browned on both sides and cooked through. Cover to keep warm

- » Meanwhile, warm cassava crepes that you will have prepared following the Cassava Crepe Recipe in the Baked goodies Section
- » Divide fish, dressing, lettuce and cucumber among tortillas and wrap to enclose your fabulous fillings

Lime buttermilk dressing Combine ingredients in small jug and stir thoroughly

Dinner Ideas

Poached Fish Cutlets with Mixed Greens Salad

Serves 4
Blood Type: all blood types
Step 1 Catabolic

Ingredients

4x7oz white fish cutlets
10cm stick fresh lemon grass, halved lengthways
1 lime, sliced thickly
Sea salt and course ground black pepper to taste (choose red chili flakes for extra zing)

Herb salad

1½oz baby asian greens
½ cup fresh coriander leaves
⅔ cup fresh mint leaves
⅓ cup fresh dill sprigs

Chili dressing

¼ cup lime juice
2 tbsp fish sauce
2 tbsp coconut oil
2 tsp xylitol
1 fresh small red thai chilli, chopped finely
1 clove garlic, chopped finely
Sea salt and course ground black pepper to taste (choose red chili flakes for extra zing)

Method

- » Place fish, lemon grass and lime in a large frying pan and barely cover the fish with cold water

»   Bring your fish slowly to a gentle simmer. Remove from heat and leave the pan to stand, covered for 10 minutes. Remove fish from the liquid and drain
»   In the meantime make your herb salad and chili dressing
»   Toss herb salad with half of the dressing
»   Serve fish topped with salad and drizzle everything with the remaining dressing

Herb Salad Combine ingredients in medium bowl

Asian Dressing Combine ingredients in screw top jar and then shake it well

Chermoula Crusted Fish

Serves 4
Blood Type: all blood types
Step 1 Catabolic

Ingredients

½ cup cassava flour
2 tbsp finely chopped fresh flat-leaf parsley
2 tbsp finely chopped fresh coriander
2 cloves garlic, crushed
1 cm piece fresh ginger, grated finely
½ tsp finely grated lemon rind
1 tsp ground cumin
1 tsp sweet paprika
1 tbsp olive oil
4x7oz white fish fillets
1 medium egg (lightly beaten)
3½oz mesclun salad greens
1 medium lemon, cut into wedges
Sea salt and course ground black pepper to taste (choose red chili flakes for extra zing)

Method

- » Preheat oven to 200°C/400°F. Oil oven tray and line with baking paper.
- » Combine cassava flour, herbs, garlic, ginger, rind, spices and oil in medium bowl.
- » Dip fish in lightly beaten egg, then in the pre made cassava breading (coat thoroughly) then place on the baking tray. Roast your fish, uncovered for about 15 minutes, or until cooked through
- » Serve fish with mesclun salad greens and lemon wedges
- » Dress with your choice of one of our fabulous dressings in our Dressings Section

Sour Fish Curry

Serves 4
Blood Type: all blood types
Step 1 Catabolic

Ingredients

1 tbsp coriander seeds
2 tsp cumin seeds
½ tsp ground turmeric
1 tsp black peppercorns
2 cm piece fresh ginger, chopped coarsely
2 cloves garlic, chopped coarsely
2 long green chillies, chopped coarsely
2 tbsp vegetable oil
4 blue-eye cutlets
2 medium brown onions, sliced thinly
1½ tsp black mustard seeds
4 fresh curry leaves
¾ cup water
⅓ cup fish stock
¼ cup lime juice
1 tbsp fish sauce
Sea salt and course ground black pepper to taste (choose red chili flakes for extra zing)

Method

- » Dry-fry the coriander and cumin seeds and turmeric in a small frying pan, stirring, until it becomes fragrant
- » Using a mortar and pestle, crush spices including peppercorns, ginger, garlic and chili to form a paste
- » Heat half of the oil in large frying pan and cook fish, uncovered, until browned on both sides. Remove from pan and cover to keep warm
- » Heat the remaining oil in same pan and cook onions, mustard seeds and curry leaves, stirring for about 5 minutes or until the onions are browned lightly

- » Add the spice paste and cook, stirring, until it all becomes fragrant again. Add water, stock, juice and sauce and bring to a boil
- » Return fish to pan and simmer, covered for about 5 minutes or until cooked as desired

Chicken in Yogurt

Serves 4
Blood Type: O, A
Step 1 Anabolic

Ingredients

2 tsp ground cumin
2 tsp ground cardamom
1 tsp ground cinnamon
½ tsp ground clove
½ tsp ground turmeric
½ cup blanched almonds
2 cm piece fresh ginger, chopped coarsely
2 cloves garlic, quartered
17½oz yogurt
8 chicken thigh cutlets (56oz), skin removed
2 tbsp vegetable oil
2 medium brown onions (10½oz), sliced thinly
⅓ cup lemon juice
¼ cup finely chopped fresh coriander
Sea salt and course ground black pepper to taste (choose red chili flakes for extra zing)

Method

- » Dry-fry spices and nuts in a small heated frying pan, stirring until the nuts are browned lightly
- » Blend or food process the nut mixture, ginger and garlic until it forms a paste
- » Combine mixture with yogurt in a large bowl, add chicken and mix all of ingredients well
- » Cover and refrigerate for at least 3 hours or overnight
- » Heat oil in large saucepan and cook onions, stirring until they are soft
- » Add the chicken mixture and simmer, covered, about 30 minutes or until chicken is cooked through. Stir in the juice
- » Serve curry sprinkled with coriander.

Lamb Curry

Serves 4
Blood Type: O, B
Step 1 Anabolic

Ingredients

1½ tbsp olive oil
35oz lamb shoulder, trimmed, diced into 3cm pieces
7oz brown onion, chopped finely
4 cloves garlic, crushed
2 tsp ground turmeric
½ tsp ground nutmeg
½ tsp ground cinnamon
½ tsp cayenne pepper
14oz can chopped tomatoes
2 cups beef stock
12oz spinach
1 tbsp finely grated lemon rind
⅓ cup toasted slivered almonds
Sea salt and course ground black pepper to taste (choose red chili flakes for extra zing)

Method

- » Heat half the oil in a large saucepan and cook lamb in batches, until browned all over
- » Heat remaining oil in same pan and cook the onions, garlic and spices, stirring, until the onion softens
- » Add lamb, un-drained tomatoes and stock then simmer, covered for about 1 hour
- » Uncover and simmer for 15 minutes or until the sauce thickens and lamb is tender
- » Add spinach and rind, stir over the heat for about 1 minute or until spinach wilts
- » Serve curry sprinkled with some sliced roasted almonds

Turkey Mince Stir Fry with Cranberries

Serves 4
Blood Type: all blood types
Step 1 Anabolic

Ingredients

1 tbsp olive oil
1 clove garlic, crushed
1 shallot, chopped finely
1 tbsp dried cranberries, chopped coarsely
7oz turkey mince
1 tbsp tamari sauce
½ tsp fish sauce
1 tbsp kecap manis (not on Step 1)
½ tsp five spice powder
1 small carrot, grated finely
1 cup finely shredded wombok (Chinese Cabbage)
2oz Lebanese cucumber, seeded, sliced thinly
1 fresh long chilli, sliced thinly
Sea salt and course ground black pepper to taste (choose red chili flakes for extra zing)
1 lime wedge

Method

- » Heat oil in a wok or deep frying pan and stir-fry the garlic, shallots and cranberries until the shallots are tender
- » Add mince and stir-fry until the mince changes color
- » Add all sauces, five spice, carrot and wombok then stir-fry until the wombok wilts (season further to taste)
- » Serve the turkey mince stir-fry topped with cucumber, chili and lime

Lemon Chicken with Greens

Serves 4
Blood Type: O, A
Step 1 Anabolic

Ingredients

2 tbsp coconut oil
17½oz chicken thigh fillets, sliced thinly
10cm stick fresh lemon grass, chopped finely
3 cloves garlic, crushed
21oz gai lan, (Chinese Broccoli or Kale) trimmed, cut into 5 cm lengths
5oz yellow capsicum, sliced thinly
2 tbsp lemon juice
2 tbsp tamari sauce
Sea salt and course ground black pepper to taste (choose red chili flakes for extra zing)

Method

- » Heat half of the oil in a wok or deep frying pan and stir-fry chicken in batches, until browned, remove from wok
- » Heat the remaining oil in the wok or deep frying pan and stir-fry lemon grass and garlic until it becomes fragrant
- » Add gai lan, capsicum, juice and sauce and stir-fry until all vegetables are tender
- » Return chicken to wok and stir-fry again until hot then season to taste

Delicious Sides

Garbanzo Bean Salad

Serves 8
Blood Type: all blood types
Step 1 Catabolic

Ingredients

1½ cups dried garbanzo beans
8½ cherry tomatoes, halved
14oz green cucumber, seeded chopped coarsely
5½oz red onion, chopped finely
¼ cup finely shredded fresh mint leaves
¼ cup lime juice
¼ cup olive oil
2 tsp Dijon mustard (natural and unsweetened)
¼ tsp xylitol
2 cloves garlic, crushed
Sea salt and course ground black pepper to taste (choose red chili flakes for extra zing)

Method

- » Place chickpeas in large bowl and cover with water. Soak overnight and drain
- » Cook chickpeas in large saucepan of boiling water, uncovered for about 50 minutes or until tender, drain. Rinse under cold water and drain again
- » Combine chickpeas in large bowl with tomato, cucumber, onion and mint, toss gently with combined remaining ingredients. Deliciously easy!

Roasted Pumpkin with Sesame Seeds

Serves 4
Blood Type: all blood types
Step 1 Anabolic

Ingredients

21oz trimmed pumpkin
Coconut Oil spray
1 tbsp agave syrup
1 tbsp sesame seeds
17½ oz asparagus, halved
5oz baby rocket leaves
3½oz red onion, sliced thinly
1 tbsp sesame oil
1 tbsp cider vinegar
1 tsp agave syrup, extra
Sea salt and course ground black pepper to taste (choose red chili flakes for extra zing)

Method

- » Preheat oven to 200°C/400°F
- » Cut pumpkin into 1.5cm wide strips. Place strips in single layer on baking-paper-lined dish and spray lightly with Coconut Oil spray
- » Lightly sprinkle fine sea salt and pepper
- » Roast, uncovered in very hot oven for about 20 minutes or until the pumpkin is just tender
- » Drizzle with agave and sprinkle with sesame seeds. Roast for a further 5 minutes, uncovered, or until the sesame seeds are browned lightly
- » In the meantime boil or steam asparagus until just tender and drain. Rinse under cold water and drain again
- » Combine pumpkin, asparagus, rocket and onion in large bowl and drizzle with the combined remaining ingredients, toss salad gently and serve

Lady's Fingers in Spicy Tomatoes

Serves 4
Blood Type: all blood types
Step 1 Catabolic

Ingredients

5 cloves garlic, quartered
2½oz shallots, chopped coarsely
2 fresh long red chilies, chopped coarsely
2 green onions, chopped finely
⅓ cup natural and unsweetened tamarind concentrate
1 tbsp vegetable oil
14oz can coconut milk
2 tbsp lime juice
10 fresh curry leaves
17½oz fresh okra, halved lengthways
14oz can crushed tomatoes
Sea salt and course ground black pepper to taste (choose red chili flakes for extra zing)

Method

- » Using a blender or food processer, blend garlic, shallots, chili, onion and tamarind until smooth
- » Heat oil in large saucepan and add tamarind mixture. Cook, stirring for about 2 minutes
- » Add coconut milk, juice and curry leaves, simmer uncovered for 5 minutes
- » Add okra and un-drained tomatoes, let simmer, uncovered for about 10 minutes or until okra is tender with still a hint of crunch

Curried Cauliflower

Serves 4
Blood Type: all blood types
Step 1 Anabolic

Ingredients

21oz cauliflower florets
2 tbsp ghee
5oz brown onion, chopped finely
2 cloves garlic, crushed
2 cm piece fresh ginger, grated
¼ cup hot curry paste
¾ cup cream
15oz tomatoes, chopped coarsely
1 cup frozen peas
1 cup yogurt
3 hard-boiled eggs, sliced thinly
¼ cup finely chopped fresh coriander
Sea salt and course ground black pepper to taste (choose red chili flakes for extra zing)

Method

- » Boil or steam cauliflower until it is just tender and drain
- » In the meantime heat ghee in large saucepan and cook onion, garlic and ginger stirring until the onion softens
- » Add paste and cook, stirring, until the mixture becomes fragrant
- » Add cream and bring to a boil then reduce heat. Add cauliflower and tomato, simmer uncovered for 5 minutes, stirring occasionally
- » Add peas and yogurt then stir over low heat for about 5 minutes or until peas are just cooked. Serve this side dish sprinkled with egg and coriander

Green Beans with Walnuts

Serves 8
Blood Type: all blood types
Step 1 Catabolic

Ingredients

8oz shallots, peeled and sliced into thin rings
½ cup olive oil
32oz green beans, trimmed
3 tbsp apple cider vinegar
3 tbsp natural and unsweetened Dijon mustard
3 tbsp olive oil
3 tbsp agave nectar **(use xylitol on Step 1)**
1 cup toasted chopped walnuts (pecans)

Method

- » Spread shallot rings on paper towel and sprinkle with salt. Cover with another paper towel and let this stand for 10 minutes. Use the paper towels to blot any excess moisture
- » Heat oil in small saucepan over a medium heat. Add shallots, and fry for 2 to 4 minutes, or until golden brown, stirring frequently
- » Pour shallots and oil through a fine mesh strainer, or remove shallots with slotted spoon
- » Spread shallots on paper towels to drain and cool. Discard the oil. Store shallots in jar, if drained
- » Cook green beans in a large pot of boiling salted water for 5 to 8 minutes, or until just tender then drain
- » Whisk together vinegar, mustard, oil and agave syrup in a serving bowl
- » Add green beans, and toss to coat everything thoroughly. Season the dish with salt and pepper, if desired
- » Top this brilliant side with the crispy shallot rings and chopped walnuts, and serve

Garlicky Brussel Sprouts

Serves 6
Blood Type: all blood types
Step 1 Catabolic

Ingredients

16oz Brussels sprouts, ends trimmed
2 tbsp olive oil
12 cloves garlic, peeled and quartered
1 tbsp xylitol
½ tsp salt
⅛ tsp ground black pepper
1 tbsp apple cider vinegar

Method

- Place brussel sprouts in a blender or food processor. Pulse for 12 to 15 minutes, or until shredded
- Heat oil in large non-stick pan over a medium-low heat then add garlic, cook for 5 to 7 minutes, or until light brown
- Increase heat to medium-high, add shredded brussel sprouts, xylitol, salt, and pepper.
- Cook for a further 5 minutes, or until they have browned, stirring often
- Add 1½ cups water, and cook 5 minutes more, or until most of liquid is evaporated. Stir in vinegar, and serve immediately

Sesame Seasoned Spinach

Serves 4
Blood Type: all blood types
Step 1 Anabolic (p.m)/Catabolic (a.m)

Ingredients

¼ cup water
16oz baby spinach
1 tbsp toasted sesame seeds
2 tsp tamari sauce
2 tsp toasted sesame oil
1 small clove garlic, minced

Method

- Place water in large pot, bring to a boil over a high heat
- Add spinach and cook, stirring frequently until the spinach has wilted about 2 to 3 minute
- Transfer to a colander and let stand until it is cool enough to handle. Squeeze out any excess water
- Coarsely chop spinach. Place in a bowl and mix in toasted sesame seeds, tamari sauce, sesame oil and garlic
- Serve at room temperature

The Carbohdrate Content

Classic Yam Puree

Serves 6
Blood Type: All blood types
Step 1 (anti fungal) Anabolic

Ingredients

60oz yam
8oz sour cream
1 cup mozzarella cheese
Juice of 1 orange (**not on Step 1**)
¼ cup salted butter
½ cup cooking cream
2 pinches of nutmeg
Sea salt and course ground black pepper to taste (choose red chili flakes for extra zing)

Method

- Peel and boil yam until soft
- Drain thoroughly and add sour cream, cooking cream, butter, nutmeg, orange juice and salt and pepper. **Add low fat milk instead of orange if on Step 1**
- For chunky mash use a masher or for a smoother puree use an electric mixer on low
- Once the desired consistency is reached transfer the puree into a baking dish, top with mozzarella and a light dusting of nutmeg
- Bake on a medium heat until cheese appears golden
- Slice into squares to create the perfect size serving to compliment your meal

Scalloped Sweet Potatoes

Serves 6
Blood Type: All blood types
Step 2 Anabolic (replace sweet potato with yam for Step 1)

Ingredients

60oz sweet potatoes or yam
½ cup fresh cooking cream
6-8oz of grated mozzarella cheese
1 tsp of mustard (unsweetened & natural)
½ tsp fine herbs or herbs of your choice
2 tsp of tapioca flour
2 tbsp of soft butter
Paprika (for topping)
Sea salt and course ground black pepper to taste (choose red chili flakes for extra zing)

Method

- » Peel and thinly slice sweet potatoes or yam and boil until nearly fully cooked, then drain
- » Melt the butter and combine the tapioca over a low heat, while stirring
- » While stirring gently add all of the cooking cream, then add cheese in small amounts,
- » Add herbs, salt and pepper until a well blended sauce is formed
- » Place all thinly sliced sweet potato or yam into a baking dish and drizzle the blended cream sauce over the entire contents being sure that it covers all of the potato or yam
- » Top the dish with a fine layer of mozzarella cheese and an even sprinkling of ground paprika
- » Bake the contents on a medium heat for 20 minutes or until top goes golden brown
- » Slice into squares to create the perfect size serving to compliment your meal

Rosemary Roasted Ground Provisions

Serves 6
Blood Type: All blood types
Step 1 (anti fungal) Anabolic

Ingredients

6oz yam/cassava
6oz butternut squash
6oz beetroot
6oz carrots
6oz parsnips (**not on Step 1**)
¼ cup olive oil
1 lemon
Sea salt and course ground black pepper to taste (choose red chili flakes for extra zing)

Method

- » Pre-heat oven to 200°C/400°F
- » Peel all veggies and slice into nice roasting sizes
- » Boil in salted water for 5-7 minutes and drain
- » Lightly oil a large baking tray and gently toss all ground provisions salt, pepper and rosemary
- » Squeeze lemon over the lot
- » Roast, occasionally tossing vegetables for about 40 minutes or until veggies are golden with a slight crisp on the outside while tender on the inside

Cassava & Parsnip Mash with Sun-Dried Tomatoes

Serves 6
Blood Type: All blood types
Step 2 Anabolic (can be Step 1 without the parsnips)

Ingredients

32oz cassava
16oz parsnips
2 teaspoons of chives
¼ cup butter
8oz sour cream
½ cup cooking cream
1 cup grated mozzarella cheese
½ cup sun-dried tomatoes
Paprika
Sea salt and course ground black pepper to taste (choose red chili flakes for extra zing)

Method

- » Peel and slice parsnips
- » Put in large saucepan and bring to a boil
- » If fresh, peel the cassava, if frozen bring to boil along with the parsnips
- » Once both ground provisions are nice and tender, drain and mash thoroughly adding the chives, butter, sour cream salt and pepper
- » Place in a baking dish, top with grated mozzarella and sprinkle paprika over the top and bake until the top is a wonderful golden colour
- » Slice into squares to create the perfect size serving to compliment your meal

Pumpkin & Yam Puree

Serves 6
Blood Type: All blood types
Step 1 (anti fungal) Anabolic

Ingredients

12oz pumpkin
12oz yam
¼ cup butter
8 oz sour cream
pinch of cinnamon
Sea salt and course ground black pepper to taste (choose red chili flakes for extra zing)

Method

- » Peel yam and pumpkin, bring to a boil in large saucepan
- » Once completely tender drain and puree using an electric mixer on low with butter, sour cream, cinnamon, salt and pepper
- » Your dish is ready to serve

Fried Cassava Chips

Serves 6
Blood Type: All blood types
Step 1 (anti fungal) Anabolic

Ingredients

32oz cassava
Olive oil
Sea salt and course ground black pepper to taste (choose red chili flakes for extra zing)

Method

- » Bring cassava to a boil and cook until tender, remembering they are then to be fried
- » Once tender, drain and toss lightly with olive oil, salt and pepper
- » Heat a shallow frying pan, and coat with olive oil
- » Once oil is hot, add cassava to pan
- » Turn them frequently and keep frying until they are golden brown and crispy
- » Your dish is ready to serve

Stocks

Beef

Makes 4 cups
Blood Type: O, B
Step 1 Anabolic

Ingredients

8oz meaty beef bones
2 medium brown onions (300g), chopped coarsely
2 trimmed celery stalks (200g), chopped coarsely
2 medium carrots (240g), chopped coarsely
3 bay leaves
2 tsp black peppercorns
2 tsp sea salt
5 cups water

Method

- Combine all ingredients in a large stock pot, bring to a boil
- Reduce heat, cover and simmer for about 1½ hours
- Strain stock into heatproof bowl; discard solids
- Allow stock to cool, cover and refrigerate

Chicken

Makes 4 cups
Blood Type: O, A
Step 1 Anabolic

Ingredients

8oz meaty chicken bones
2 medium onions (300g), chopped coarsely
2 trimmed celery stalks (200g), chopped coarsely
2 medium carrots (240g), chopped coarsely
3 bay leaves
2 tsp black peppercorns
2 tsp sea salt
4 cups water

Method

- » Combine all ingredients in a large stock pot, bring to a boil
- » Reduce heat, cover and simmer for about 1½ hours
- » Strain stock into heatproof bowl; discard solids
- » Allow stock to cool, cover and refrigerate

Fish

Makes 4 cups
Blood Type: all blood types
Step 1 Catabolic

Ingredients

8oz fish bones
2 medium onion (300g), chopped coarsely
2 trimnmed celery stalks (200g), chopped coarsely
2 medium carrots (240g), chopped coarsely
3 bay leaves
2 tsp black peppercorns
2 tsp sea salt
5 cups water

Method

- » Combine all ingredients in a large stock pot, bring to a boil
- » Reduce heat, cover and simmer for about 1½ hours
- » Strain stock into heatproof bowl; discard solids
- » Allow stock to cool, cover and refrigerate

Vegetable

Makes 4 cups
Blood Type: all blood types
Step 1 Anabolic

Ingredients

2 large carrots (360g), chopped coarsely
4 medium onions (600g), chopped coarsely
10 trimmed celery stalks (1kg), chopped coarsely
2 large sweet peppers (250g), chopped coarsely
4 bay leaves
2 tsp black peppercorns
2 tsp sea salt
5 cups water

Method

- » Combine all ingredients in a large stock pot, bring to a boil
- » Reduce heat, cover and simmer for about 1½ hours
- » Strain stock into heatproof bowl; discard solids
- » Allow stock to cool, cover and refrigerate

Soups

Creamy Soup

Serves 4
Blood Type: all blood types
Step 1 Anabolic (p.m)/Catabolic (a.m)

Ingredients

1.5oz butter
3½ oz onion, chopped finely
1 clove garlic, crushed
4½oz turkey, chopped finely
2 tbsp cassava flour
14oz yam, chopped coarsely
3 cups cooking cream
2 cups vegetable stock
14oz firm white fish fillets, chopped coarsely
2 tbsp fresh chives, finely chopped
2 tbsp fresh thyme, finely chopped
2tbsp fresh coriander, finely chopped
2 pinches of ground cumin
Sea salt and course ground black pepper to taste (choose red chili flakes for extra zing)

Method

- » Melt the butter in a large saucepan. Cook the onions, garlic, and turkey, until the onion softens.
- » Add flour and stir in then let sit for 1 minute
- » Add yam, cream, stock and fresh herbs and bring to a boil
- » Reduce heat and simmer covered for about 15-20 minutes or until yam is tender

- » Add fish and simmer uncovered for about 4 minutes or until the fish is cooked through
- » Salt and pepper to taste

Chicken a la Coconut

Serves 4
Blood Type: O, A
Step 1 Anabolic

Ingredients

1 tbsp coconut oil
21oz chicken thigh fillets, cut into 1cm strips
¼ cup green curry paste
4 cups chicken stock (natural and unsweetened)
3¼ cups coconut milk
1 long green chilli, chopped finely
8 fresh kaffir lime leaves, shredded
4oz rice vermicelli **(not on Step 1)**
2 tbsp xylitol
2 tbsp lime juice
2 tbsp fish sauce
1 cup bean sprouts
½ cup mint leaves
1 long green chilli, sliced thinly
2 limes cut into thin wedges
Sea salt and course ground black pepper to taste (choose red chili flakes for extra zing)

Method

- Heat oil in large saucepan and cook chicken in batches until it has lightly browned
- Add paste to same pan and gently stir around until it becomes fragrant
- Return chicken to pan with stock, coconut milk, chopped chili and lime leaf and bring to a boil
- Reduce heat and simmer uncovered for 30 minutes, gently skimming fat from the surface occasionally

- » Add vermicelli and cook, uncovered until just tender. Stir in xylitol, juice and sauce. (The vermicelli can be prepared separately for those on Step 1)
- » Serve your fragrant soup sprinkled with sprouts, mint, sliced chili and lime.

Beef Pho

Serves 6
Blood Type: O, B
Step 2 Anabolic

Ingredients

8 cups water
4 cups beef stock (natural and unsweetened)
1 kg chuck steak
2 star anise
1oz fresh ginger, grated
⅓ cup tamari sauce
7oz bean thread noodles **(not on Step 1)**
1½ cups bean sprouts
¼ cup coriander leaves
⅓ cup fresh mint leaves
4 green onions, sliced thinly
2 fresh long red chillies, sliced thinly
¼ cup fish sauce
1 medium lemon, (5oz) cut into 6 wedges
Sea salt and course ground black pepper to taste (choose red chili flakes for extra zing)

Method

- » Place water and stock in large saucepan with beef, star anise, ginger and tamari sauce, bring to a boil
- » Reduce heat and simmer, covered for 30 minutes. Uncover and simmer for about 30 minutes or until beef is tender
- » Meanwhile, place noodles in medium heatproof bowl, cover with boiling water and stand until they are just tender then drain
- » Combine sprouts, coriander, mint, onion, and chili in a medium bowl
- » Remove beef from pan, strain the broth into a large heatproof bowl and discard the solids

- » When beef is cool enough to handle, remove and discard the fat and sinew
- » Slice beef thinly and return to same cleaned pan with broth and bring to a boil. Then slowly stir in the fish sauce
- » Divide noodles among the soup bowls, ladle hot beef broth into bowls, sprinkle with prepared sprout mixture and serve with lemon

Gazpacho

Serves 4
Blood Type: all blood types
Step 1 Catabolic

Ingredients

3 cups natural and unsweetened tomato juice
8 medium egg tomatoes, chopped coarsely
6oz red onion, chopped coarsely
1 clove garlic, quartered
4½oz cucumber, chopped coarsely
5oz red capsicum, chopped coarsely
2 tsp tabasco sauce
4 green onions, chopped finely
2oz cucumber, seeded, chopped finely
2½oz yellow capsicum, chopped finely
2 tsp olive oil
1 tbsp vodka (only step 2)
2 tbsp finely chopped fresh coriander
Sea salt and course ground black pepper to taste (choose red chili flakes for extra zing)

Method

- » Blend or process juice, tomatoes, red onions, garlic, chopped cucumbers and red capsicum, in batches until pureed
- » Strain the mixture through a sieve into large bowl, then cover and refrigerate 3 hours
- » Combine remaining ingredients in a small bowl.
- » Serve your bowls of soup topped with the delicious vegetable mixture.

Chilled Cucumber

Serves 4
Blood Type: all blood types
Step 1 Catabolic

Ingredients

18oz cucumbers, peeled, grated coarsely
1 clove garlic, quartered
1 tbsp lemon juice
1 tbsp coarsely chopped fresh mint
17½oz greek-style yogurt
Sea salt and course ground black pepper to taste (choose red chili flakes for extra zing)

Method

- » Place cucumbers in a sieve over a bowl, cover and refrigerate for at least 3 hours or overnight. Reserve the cucumber liquid in bowl, squeeze any excess liquid from the cucumbers
- » Blend or food process cucumbers, garlic, juice and mint until mixture is smooth and transfer to large bowl
- » Stir yogurt into cucumber mixture and add the reserved cucumber liquid, a little at a time, stirring until soup is of the desired consistency
- » Serve bowls of soup topped with extra mint and toasted cassava bread (see Cassava Bread recipe in Baked Goods section)

Curried Cauliflower Soup

Serves 6
Blood Type: all blood types
Step 1 Catabolic

Ingredients

1 tbsp olive oil
5oz brown onion, chopped finely
2 cloves garlic
½ cup mild curry paste
8 cups water
1 small cauliflower, trimmed, chopped coarsely
14oz yam
1 tbsp tomato paste
1 cup buttermilk
½ cup loosely packed fresh coriander leaves
Sea salt and course ground black pepper to taste (choose red chili flakes for extra zing)

Method

- » Heat oil in a large saucepan and cook onions and garlic, stirring, until onion softens
- » Add curry paste and cook, stirring for around 5 minutes
- » Add water, cauliflower, potato and tomato paste and bring to a boil then reduce the heat and simmer uncovered for about 15 minutes or until the vegetables are tender
- » Allow to cool for 15 minutes
- » Blend or food process soup, in batches until smooth. Return soup to the same cleaned pot, add buttermilk and stir gently over a low heat until completely hot
- » Serve bowls of soup sprinkled with coriander and, if desired, accompanied with pizza squares sprinkled with hot olive oil and garlic then baked. (see The Pizza Crust Recipe in The Baked Goodies Section)

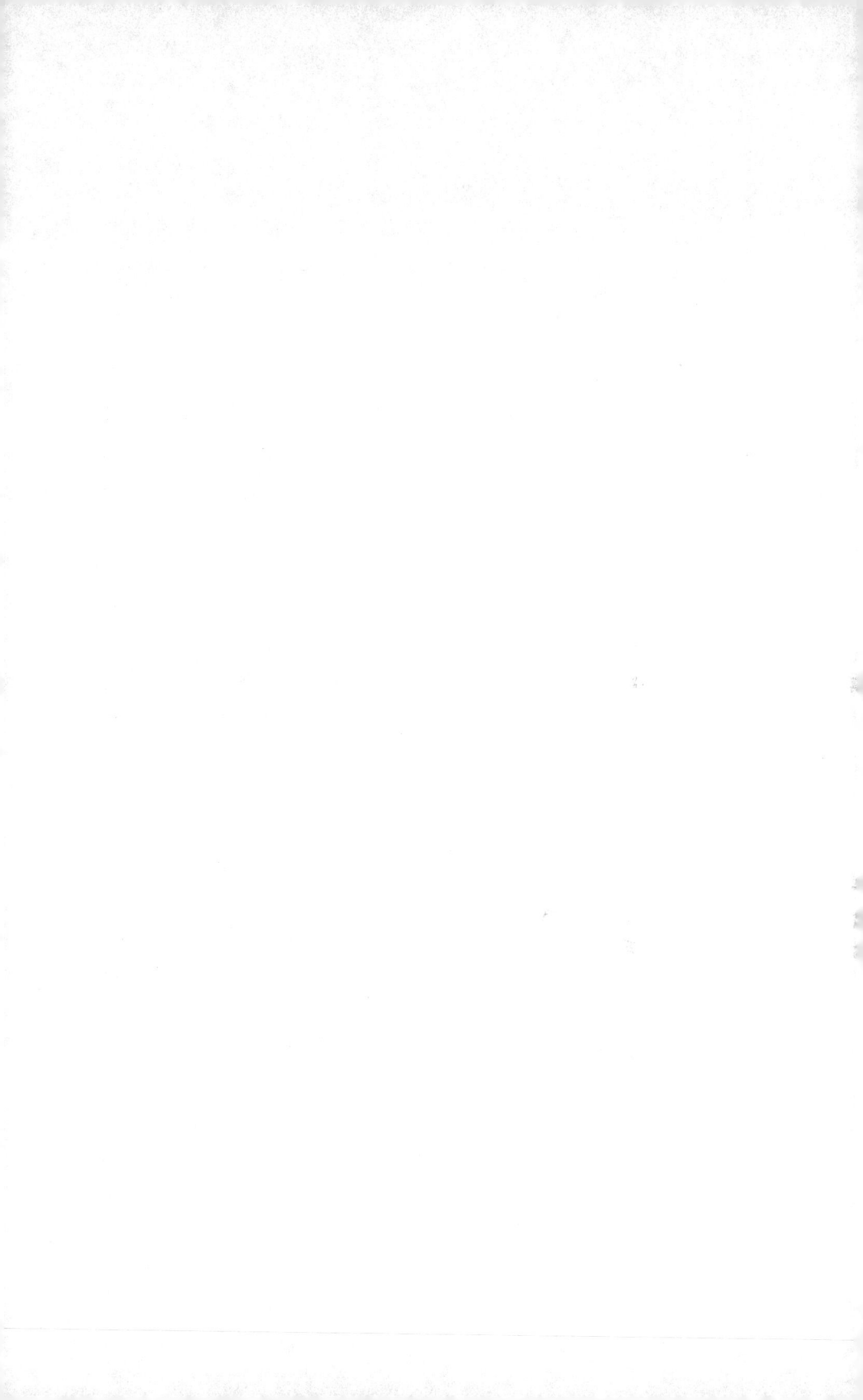